EATING
FOR
RESULTS

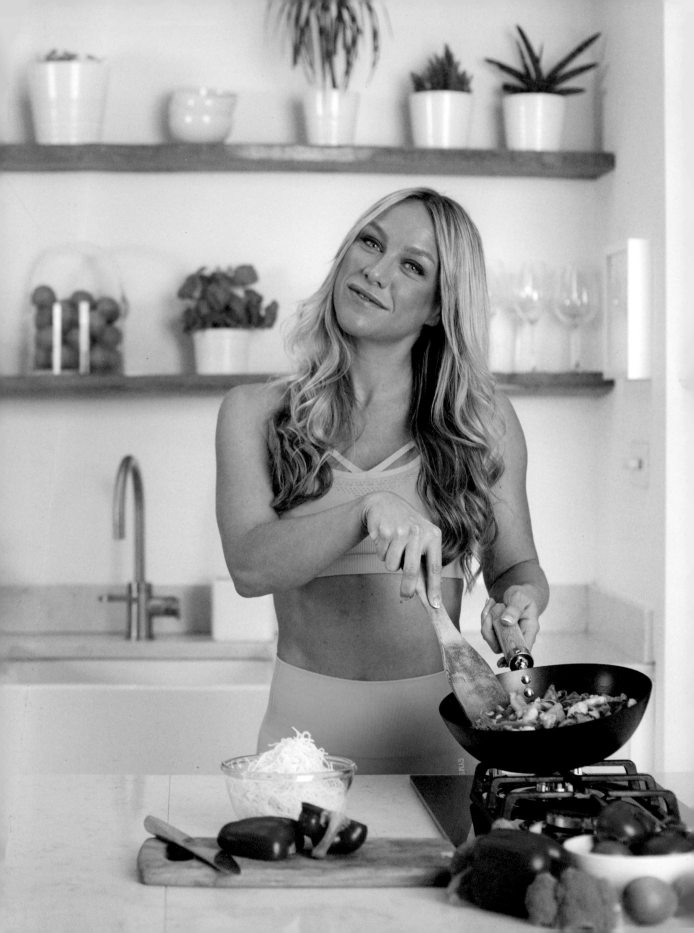

EATING FOR RESULTS
CHLOE MADELEY

Delicious, easy recipes to help you reach
your health and fitness goal

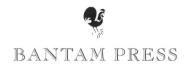

BANTAM PRESS

LONDON · NEW YORK · TORONTO · SYDNEY · AUCKLAND

TRANSWORLD PUBLISHERS
Penguin Random House, One Embassy Gardens,
8 Viaduct Gardens, London SW11 7BW

Transworld is part of the Penguin Random House group of companies
whose addresses can be found at global.penguinrandomhouse.com

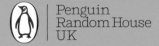
Penguin
Random House
UK

First published in Great Britain in 2020 by Bantam Press
an imprint of Transworld Publishers

A CIP catalogue record for this book is available from the British Library.

ISBN 9781787631618

Project editor: Jo Roberts-Miller
Design: Smith & Gilmour
Cover and exercise photography by Sam Riley
Food photography by Smith & Gilmour
Food styling: Phil Mundy
Chloe's hair and makeup by Meera Shah

Typeset in Museo Slab 9.75/14pt by Smith & Gilmour
Printed in China by Toppan Leefung Printing Ltd

The information in this book has been compiled by way of general
guidance to the specific subjects addressed. It is not a substitute and not to
be relied on for medical advice. Please consult your GP before making any
significant diet or lifestyle changes that may affect your health. So far as the
author is aware the information given is correct and up to date at the time
of publication. The author and publishers disclaim, as far as the law allows,
any liability arising directly or indirectly from the use, or misuse, of the
information contained in this book.

Penguin Random House is committed to a sustainable
future for our business, our readers and our planet. This book
is made from Forest Stewardship Council® certified paper.

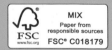

1 3 5 7 9 10 8 6 4 2

CONTENTS

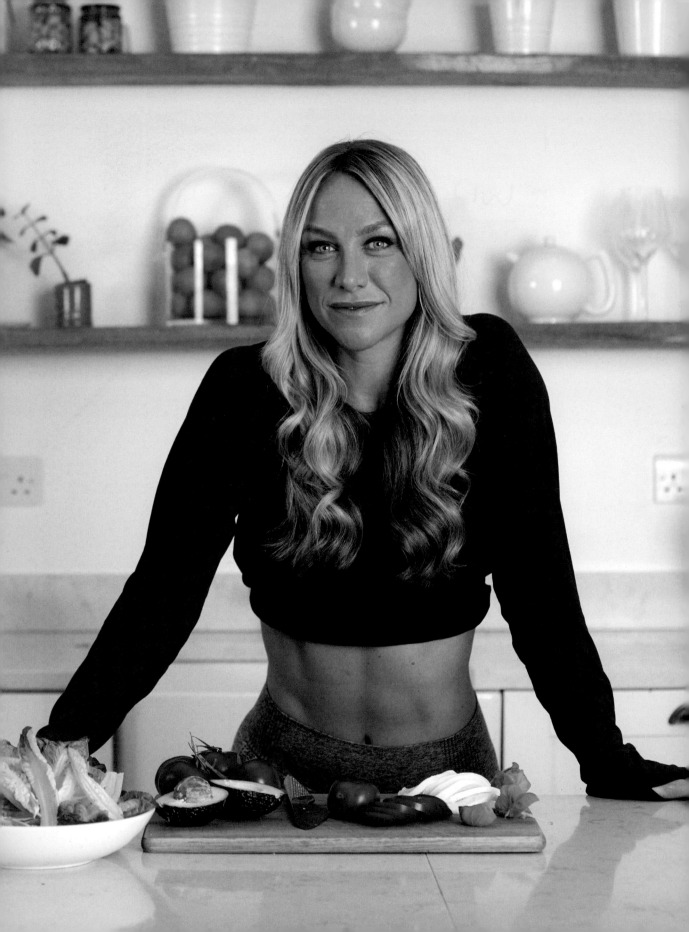

INTRODUCTION

When I first decided to work in health and fitness, it was solely because I had fallen in love with weight lifting.

Less than a month later, I found myself sitting down to my 'Level 2 Gym Instruction' and 'Level 3 Personal Training' *Active IQ* courses.

As the months rolled on and I gradually began to add to my qualifications, the syllabus became more and more advanced, culminating in the final months, which were dedicated to nutrition...

Only then were my eyes opened to the paramount importance of food for the body, and to the vast amount of shockingly bad information out there.

My love for nutrition rapidly matched my love for lifting, and I have spent the last seven years trying to keep up-to-date with all things food and the body. Like all science, what we know about nutrition is ever evolving, and that's what keeps it so interesting to me.

For years I was inundated with requests from clients – both online and in person – for recipe guides and cookbooks, and while I've always loved cooking (I consider it one of my biggest passions), writing a cookbook is another thing entirely... The mere thought of it overwhelmed me, so I shied away from it.

When my first book (*The 4-Week Body Blitz*) was in the making, I realised the importance of giving readers nutritional guidance and recipe ideas alongside the exercises to ensure they got the very best results and fuelled their exercise and recovery in the right way. So I trudged off and came up with some of my own meal ideas!

And, without a doubt, the most successful chapters of all of my books to date have been the recipe guides...

And so, we come to *Eating for Results*!

You will notice that all of the recipes in this book are extremely simple and straightforward. I made a conscious effort to include ingredients that are easy to find and cheap to buy, and recipes that are easy to make and quick to cook.

This is because every time I talk about a recipe or a book of mine online, the number one question I am asked is: Are the ingredients cheap and easy to find?!

The second question I am asked is: I have an extremely busy life; is this recipe quick and easy to make?!

Like my audience, I am a massive fan of Jamie Oliver's *5 Ingredients* and Joe Wicks's *Lean in 15*. I like these books because they are simple and easy to implement for everyone.

However, *Eating for Results* serves a more specific purpose – this cookbook is a road map to the physique you've always wanted...

ABOUT THIS BOOK...

Unlike other cookbooks, *Eating for Results* is a recipe guide that will help you match your food intake to your physique and training goal.

First, you decide on your goal:
>> **Fat Loss**
>> **Muscle Building / Performance**
>> **General Health and Fitness**

Then, find your goal-appropriate recipes:

>> Lower calorie, high-protein recipes for **Fat-loss Goals**

>> Higher calorie, high-macro split recipes for **Muscle-building and / or Performance Goals**

>> Nutritious, well-balanced calorie and macro split recipes for **General Health and Fitness Goals**

To cater for your various dietary requirements and preferences, I've made sure that each goal includes recipe options that are:

 Low carb   Vegetarian

 High carb   Vegan

I have also included calorie and macro breakdowns alongside every recipe, so readers can easily track their intake and / or amend amounts to hit their own specific numbers.

There are three main sections:

1. **Breakfast and Brunch Recipes**
2. **Lunch and Dinner Recipes**
3. **Snack Recipes**

Within each section, I've ordered the recipes so that vegan and vegetarian recipes are followed by those with fish, then meat.

Every recipe is colour coded to match goal and dietary preference, and:

>> Uses **healthy** ingredients

>> Uses **minimal** ingredients

>> Is **quick and easy** to make

>> Is **tried and tested** to achieve maximum flavour

Finally, I have added meal plans at the end of the book to make it even easier for you to plan your food for the week.

A Quick Explanation of the Micro- and Macronutrients

Those of you who have my previous books will know that there are three macronutrients (nutrients our bodies **need** in order to survive and achieve optimum health):

>> **Proteins** (e.g. chicken, fish, meat, egg whites, dairy, soy, protein powders, **combined** plant-based foods)

>> **Fats** (e.g. oils, oily fish, fatty meats, egg yolks, dairy, nuts, seeds, avocados)

>> **Carbohydrates** (e.g. grains, fruit, refined sugars, starchy vegetables, legumes)

There are also other vital nutrients to consider, such as:

>> **Micronutrients** (vitamins and minerals necessary for optimum physical health, function and survival)

>> **Fibre** (a plant-based substance that is pivotal to gut health and digestion – and also very satiating, which is extremely helpful if you have a fat-loss goal)

It doesn't matter if you're a vegan, a vegetarian, a low-carb dieter or a body builder, **protein** should always be your dominant macronutrient and **micronutrients** and **fibre** should be daily dietary staples.

Protein is incredibly important because it is a macronutrient that your body *needs* in order to function on a base, cellular level. It is this macro that is responsible for the entire structure and function of the human body, and all of the tissues and organs within it.

Every recipe in this book is high in protein, including the vegan and vegetarian recipes. This is achieved by including animal proteins, combined plant-based proteins, soy, Quorn and / or protein supplements like powders.

Your body also *needs* **micronutrients** (vitamins and minerals) in order to maintain optimum health and survive. You can absorb these from wholefoods, supplements and various other lifestyle implementations. When it comes to *plant-based* wholefoods, you're also getting a good old hit of dietary **fibre**...

This is a double whammy that should be taken advantage of every day, in my opinion.

Now let's talk a bit more about the two 'energy macros'...

Fats (especially unsaturated fats, like oily fish, but also saturated fats, like red meat) play a pivotal role in your body's physical, hormonal and restorative makeup. Fats are what we call an 'energy macro' and, just like proteins, fatty acids are *essential*, meaning it is *essential* that we get them from our dietary intake...

Unlike **carbohydrates**...

Carbs have been (wrongly) demonised for a long time. It is true that *technically* they are *not* a macronutrient (meaning our bodies do not *need* them in order to survive). *However*, if you train hard and have physique or performance goals, carbs SHOULD ABSOLUTELY feature in your daily diet.

Like fats, carbohydrates are considered to be an 'energy macro' and are converted to glucose in the blood, being stored later as glycogen in the liver and muscle.

It goes without saying that if you have performance or physique goals, carbohydrates should be consumed pre- and post-workout, or on intermittent days each week at the very least.

All physique results (muscle building and / or fat loss)

and

All performance results (strength and / or fitness)

require

All of the previously listed nutrients (protein, fats and carbohydrates)...

The only difference is that each goal requires different AMOUNTS of each nutrient (the overall calorie intake and macronutrient division will be different).

In this cookbook, there are recipes for every body type, every dietary preference, and every physique goal.

A Note About the Recipes

The **Fat-loss Recipes** in this book are all HIGH in protein, but LOW in one or both of the two energy macros (fats and carbs).

This is simply to keep your calorie intake LOW (the key to a successful fat-loss diet), while allowing for a well-balanced macronutrient and energy intake throughout the day.

The **Muscle-building and Performance Recipes** in this book are all HIGH in protein and BOTH of the energy macros, but more predominantly carbohydrates.

This is simply to keep your calorie intake HIGH (the key to a successful muscle-building and / or high-performance diet), and enhance your ability to both train hard and recover well.

The **General Health and Fitness Recipes** in this book are all nicely balanced in terms of their calorie and macronutrient ratios. They are neither HIGH nor LOW in calories or macros.

This is to keep your intake nice and level, encouraging overall health, fitness, recovery and wellbeing.

The bottom line is, your calories and macros need to be in line with your goals or it's unlikely you will get anywhere at all.

A Word on Calorie Intakes

If you have body transformation goals (muscle building and / or fat loss), your diet needs to be structured around the following five factors *(listed in order of importance)* for you to be successful:

1. **Calorie intake**
2. **Macronutrient split**
3. **Specific food choices**
4. **Nutrient timing**
5. **Supplementation**

Most people know that the universally recommended calorie intake for women is 2000kcals per day. For men, it is 2500kcals per day.

Most people also know that 1lb is estimated to equal about 3500kcals.

So, for a woman to lose 1lb a week, the equation looks like this:

>> 2000kcals per day x 7 = 14,000kcals per week (maintenance)

>> 14,000kcals per week – 3500kcals = 10,500kcals per week (weight loss)

>> 10,500kcals per week / 7 = 1500kcals per day (weight loss)

This is the estimated calorie deficit for your average woman, but it's important to remember the words **estimated** and **average.** The specific numbers **can vary greatly** from woman to woman.

Please note that this works in reverse for weight / muscle gain, too – in other words: +1lb = +3500kcals per week.

How you choose to implement this deficit (or surplus) is completely up to you. Some common ways include:

>> Eating a little less than usual every day – e.g. reducing your daily intake by 500kcals (this would bring the daily total to 1500kcals for women and 2000kcals for men).

>> Implementing a weekly fast of 24–48 hours (consecutive or intermittent), which could total a deficit of between 2000–4000kcals per week.

>> Cutting out a macronutrient, such as proteins, carbs or fats (as implemented with Atkins and keto diets, for example – I do not recommend this).

>> Increasing your daily activity by 500kcals' worth of exercise.

While the above is tried and tested, as always, there is a big grey area:

>> If you are extremely active (you train like an athlete or have a manual job), you might not need to implement too much (if any) of a *dietary* deficit at all in order to get results, because you are already burning more calories than you are consuming (this is a calorie deficit achieved via activity output, not reduction of food input).

>> If you are extremely sedentary and you don't like to train or move around a lot, you might need to implement an even more extreme dietary deficit in order to see results, hovering just above your basic calorie needs.

>> These numbers are AVERAGES. I've had some female clients achieve fantastic fat loss on around 2000kcals per day, and I've had to drop some clients down to around 1200kcals per day. Different heights, weights, ages and jobs all count when determining what calories work best for YOU.

>> Our body's ability to burn calories for energy (its metabolism) varies and adapts. In other words, the longer we eat in a deficit, the more our metabolic rate slows down to match our food intake. This is a survival mechanism; your body doesn't care if you want to lose weight, it wants to SURVIVE. The good news is this also works in reverse, which is why in all of my books I recommend SLOWLY coming out of a deficit after a period of months.

ALL of the above factors mean that the best way to implement a calorie deficit is as follows:

>> Start high, monitor your weekly results and if you aren't dropping weight, you simply aren't in a deficit yet...

>> If you aren't in a deficit, drop calories by a small amount (100kcals, for example) and try again.

This will stop you from starving yourself and will allow you to learn what YOUR specific calorie intake should be.

Please note, this works in reverse for weight gain (aka muscle building).

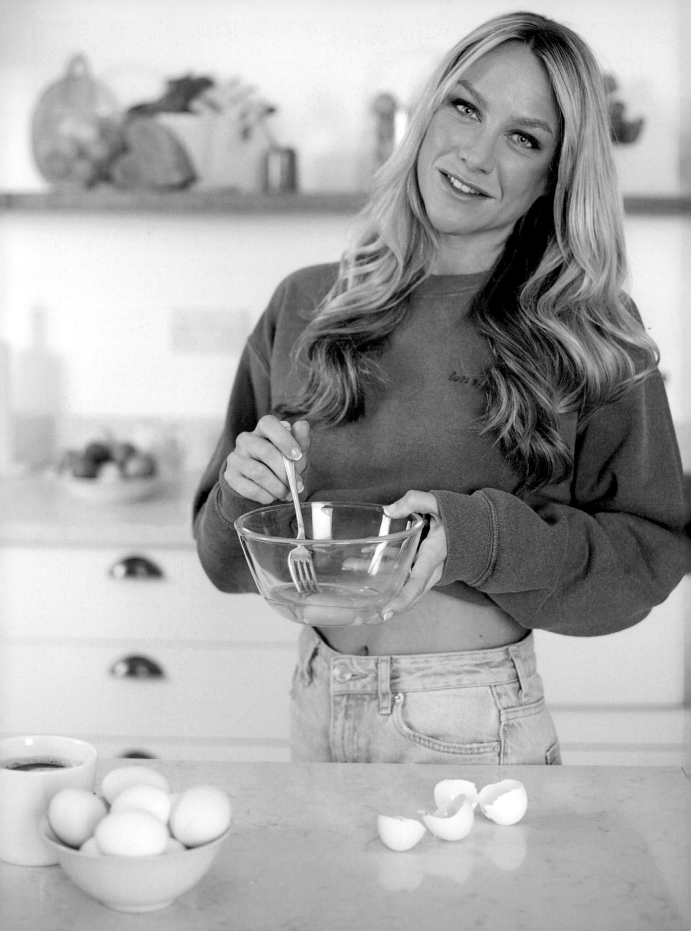

BREAKFAST AND BRUNCH

● ○ ○

These easy-to-prepare recipes are filling – they will help you get going in the morning and keep your energy levels up.

FAT-LOSS GOALS
(low-calorie and high-protein recipes)

Fat loss is only achieved when you are in a calorie **deficit** (the number of calories you consume via food needs to be smaller than the number of calories you use via movement; this is called a Negative Energy Balance).

These fat-loss recipes are ALL low in calories and high in protein, with different quantities of the two energy macros (fats and carbs), according to your preference.

*Please note: Regardless of goals, I ALWAYS recommend carbohydrate consumption pre- and post-workout. If you train in the morning, I advise you to choose a higher carb recipe both before and after your training session. If you train fasted, that's fine, just make sure to have a higher carb recipe **post**-training.*

Lean Beans on Toast

SERVES 1

Every time you see a wholegrain and a legume in this book, you're seeing a complete protein. Mixing these two food groups will ensure you get a good hit of essential amino acids.

1 rasher turkey bacon,
   roughly chopped
200g baked beans
   (homemade see page 182
   or 1 small tin – low sugar
   is best)
1 slice wholemeal bread
   (typically 40–50g)
1 tsp butter

1. Place a non-stick frying pan over a high heat, add the bacon and cook until crisp.

2. Meanwhile, place the beans in a saucepan over a medium heat. Add the crispy bacon to the beans and bring to a simmer.

3. Toast and butter the bread and put on a plate.

4. Pour the beans and bacon over the toast and serve.

This recipe is easily adapted for vegetarians by removing the bacon and replacing with one rasher of Quorn bacon, or even a small handful of tofu pieces. However, you could just remove the bacon since the combination of the wholemeal bread and the beans already forms a complete protein.

FAT-LOSS

CALORIES: 357
Protein: 18.7g
Fats: 28g
Carbs: 9.1g

Mexican Omelette

SERVES 1

Those of you with my previous books will know I love a Mexican breakfast! So far, I've had a Mexican scramble and a burrito, but here's a new spin on an old favourite.

2 small eggs
pinch paprika or chilli
    powder (optional)
1 small handful grated
    cheese
½ jalapeño pepper, sliced
½ large tomato, diced
½ small avocado, diced
1 tbsp salsa (homemade see
    page 180 or shop-bought)

1. Whisk the eggs in a small bowl and season with salt, freshly ground black pepper and the paprika or chilli powder, if using.

2. Place a non-stick frying pan over a medium heat. Pour in the egg mixture then sprinkle the grated cheese over half of the mixture and top with the jalapeño and tomato. Swirl the pan in a circular motion as the omelette cooks, so the mixture spreads and cooks evenly. Use a spatula to pull in the sides of the omelette to allow any uncooked mixture to reach the surface of the pan.

3. When the omelette is cooked to your desired consistency (I like mine a little runny but everybody is different), fold the plain half over the filled half and slide on to a plate.

4. Scatter the avocado over the omelette, spoon on the salsa and serve.

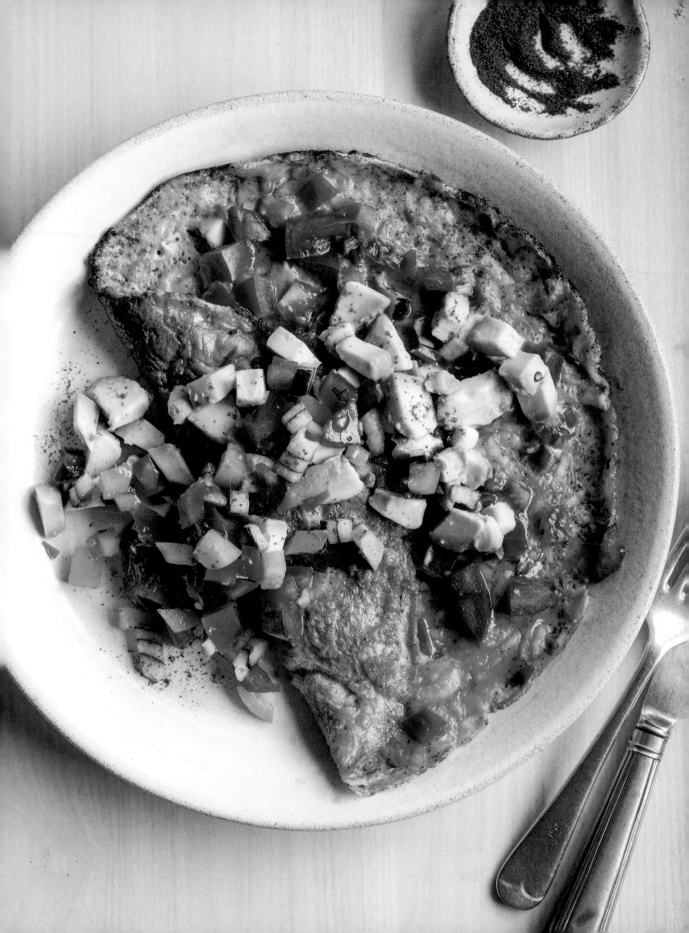

FAT-LOSS
CALORIES: 327
Protein: 30.2g
Fats: 22.5g
Carbs: 1g

Egg Bites

SERVES 1

These little beauties are perfect for bacon and egg enthusiasts. In our version we sliced 2 asparagus spears and added them before baking – see the Veggie Tip below for more veg suggestions.

3 slices Parma ham
3 small eggs
3 tsp grated cheese
1 tbsp chopped fresh
    chives, to serve (optional)

1. Preheat the oven to 200°C/Fan 180°C and line three holes of a non-stick muffin tin or three dariole moulds with the Parma ham slices.

2. Whisk the eggs in a bowl and season well with freshly ground black pepper.

3. Divide the egg mixture evenly between the Parma ham cups.

4. Drop 1 teaspoon of grated cheese into each cup and bake in the oven for 20 minutes.

5. Remove from the oven, sprinkle with chives, if using, and serve.

This recipe is easily adaptable for vegetarians simply by removing the Parma ham. You could add thin strips of avocado, diced tomato, or any veg you prefer to the egg mixture before baking. Non-veggies could add veg, too. So long as veg additions are non-starchy, you can add any you like. The same goes for herbs and spices – try roughly chopped parsley or coriander, or a pinch of paprika.

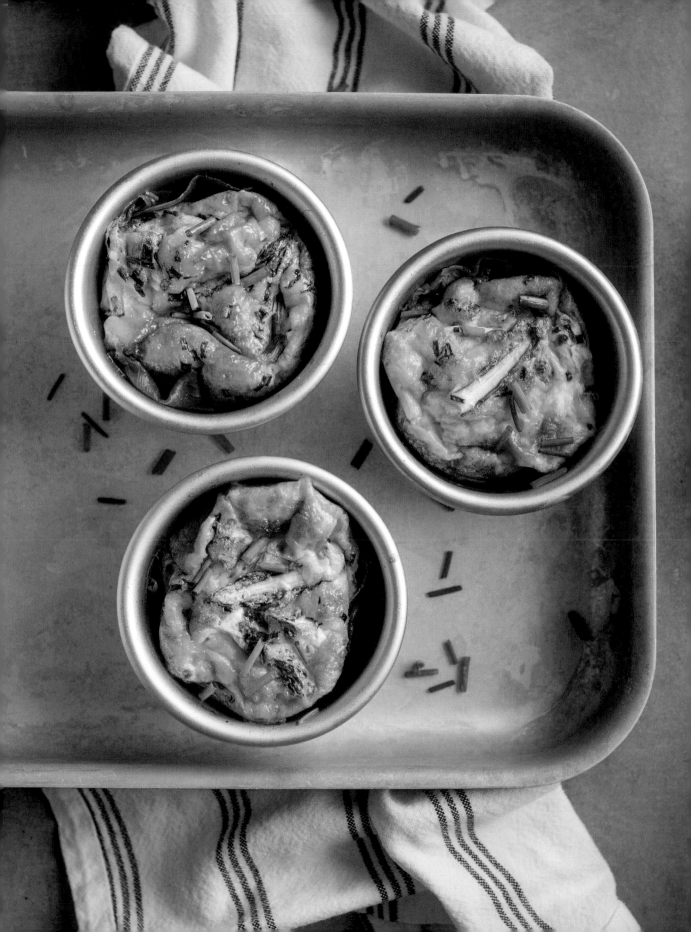

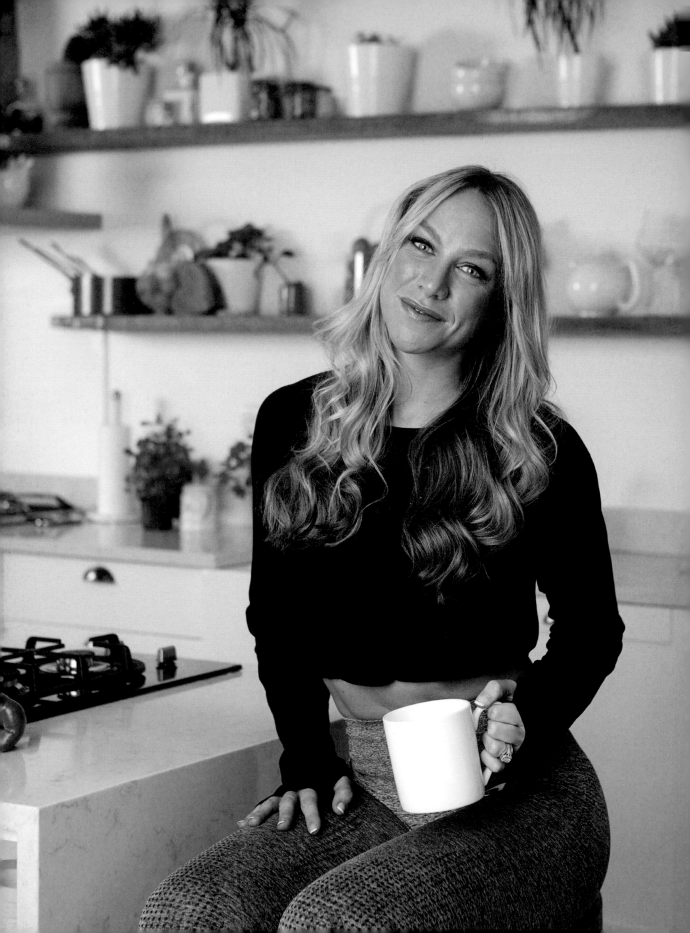

Mediterranean Scramble

SERVES 1

I usually make my scramble Mexican but eggs and basil are a match made in Mediterranean heaven!

1 large handful cherry tomatoes, halved or quartered
2 large handfuls torn mozzarella
1 handful fresh basil leaves, torn
3 small eggs

COOK'S TIP

Adding 2 slices of toast or 300g potatoes to any of the savoury fat-loss recipes would transform them into muscle-building and performance-enhancing recipes (by increasing both macro and calorie quantities).

1. Combine the cherry tomatoes, mozzarella and basil in a small bowl and set aside.

2. Beat the eggs in a separate bowl and season well with salt and freshly ground black pepper.

3. Place a non-stick frying pan over a high heat then pour the eggs into the centre.

4. Reduce the heat to low-medium and stir the eggs while they cook.

5. When they reach your desired consistency (I like my eggs slightly runny but everybody is different), stir in the tomatoes, mozzarella and basil.

6. Remove from the heat, check the seasoning and serve.

FAT-LOSS

CALORIES: 346
Protein: 35.9g
Fats: 16.9g
Carbs: 12g

Spicy Chicken Patties

SERVES 1

This is for sausage fans who are missing their indulgent breakfasts! Serve alongside a generous helping of breakfast veggies, like grilled tomatoes, mushrooms or spinach.

4 Heck chicken chipolatas
½ small onion (any),
    peeled and diced
1 jalapeño pepper, diced
1 large egg
1 tbsp grated cheese

COOK'S TIP

You can use red or white onions in this dish – my husband prefers the sweetness of red onion with sausage meat, but I like the sharpness of white.

1. Squeeze the sausage meat out of the casings and place in a mixing bowl. Add the onion and jalapeño.

2. Crack the egg into the bowl and add the cheese. Mix the ingredients together using your hands.

3. Place a non-stick frying pan over a high heat and spoon the mixture into the pan in 3 large dollops. Turn down the heat to medium and cook for approximately 3–4 minutes on each side.

4. Season with freshly ground black pepper to serve.

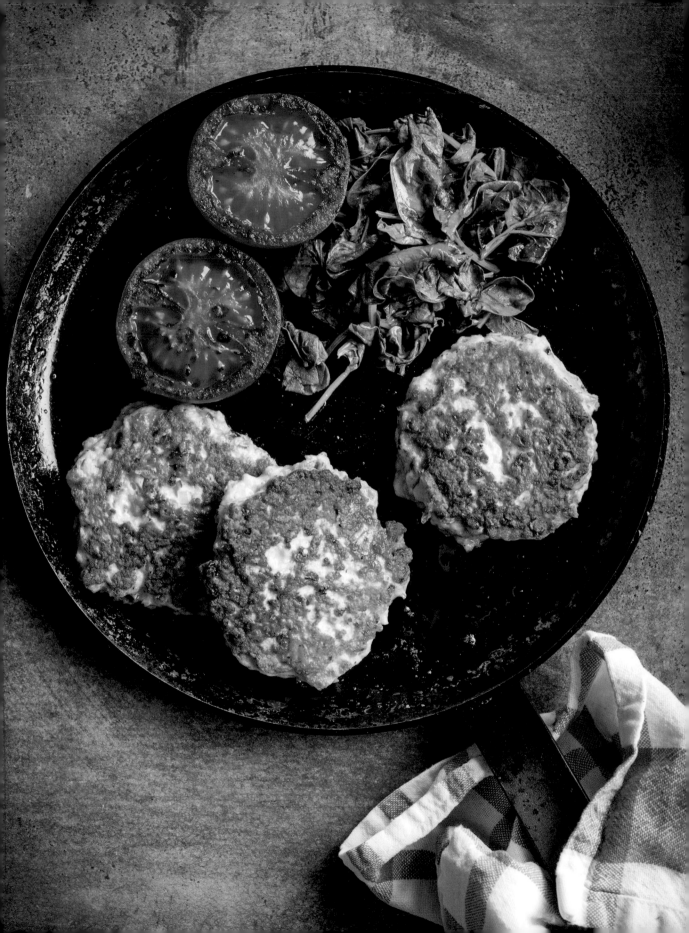

FAT-LOSS

CALORIES: 365
Protein: 23.7g
Fats: 16.7g
Carbs: 32.5g

Crunchy Banana Shake

SERVES 1

I always include a shake in my breakfast recipes because I know people don't have a lot of time in the morning. This is a great option for pre- or post-workout, too, as it's high in all three macros.

1 scoop whey or vegan protein powder
500ml unsweetened nut milk (any)
1 level tbsp crunchy nut butter
    (homemade see page 183 or
    shop-bought)
1 medium banana, peeled
1 large handful ice (optional)

1. Place all ingredients in a blender and whizz until you reach the desired consistency.

2. Pour into a glass and serve.

FAT-LOSS

CALORIES: 388
Protein: 31.5g
Fats: 6g
Carbs: 44g

The Lean Greens Shake

SERVES 1

An incredibly healthy way to start your day!

1 small green apple, cored and
    roughly chopped
1 small kiwi fruit, peeled and
    roughly chopped
1 mini cucumber, roughly chopped
1 small stick celery, roughly chopped
1 small pot 0% Greek (or soy) yoghurt
    (approx. 170g)
500ml light and / or unsweetened soy milk
1 large handful ice (optional)

1. Place all ingredients in a blender and whizz until you reach the desired consistency.

2. Pour into a glass to serve.

This recipe is easily adaptable for vegans simply by using soy yoghurt instead of Greek yoghurt.

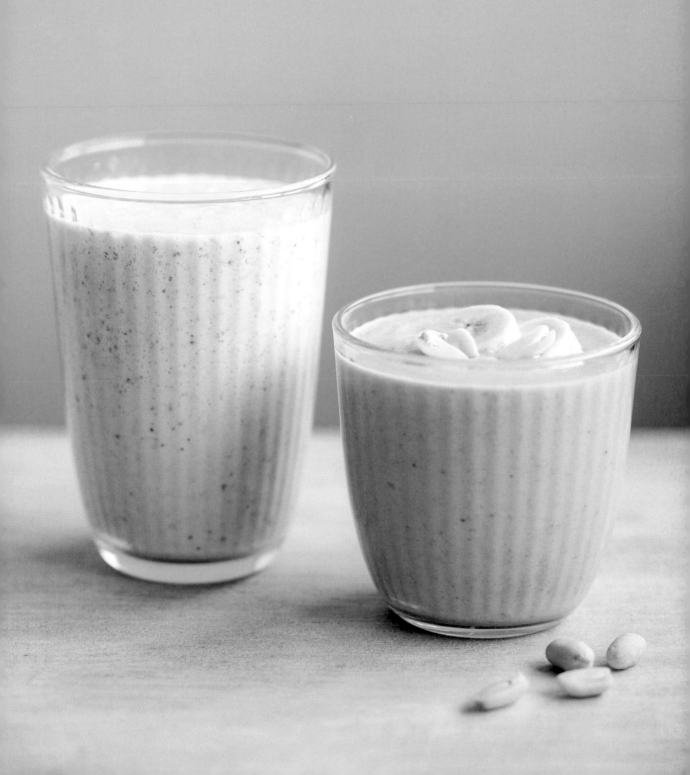

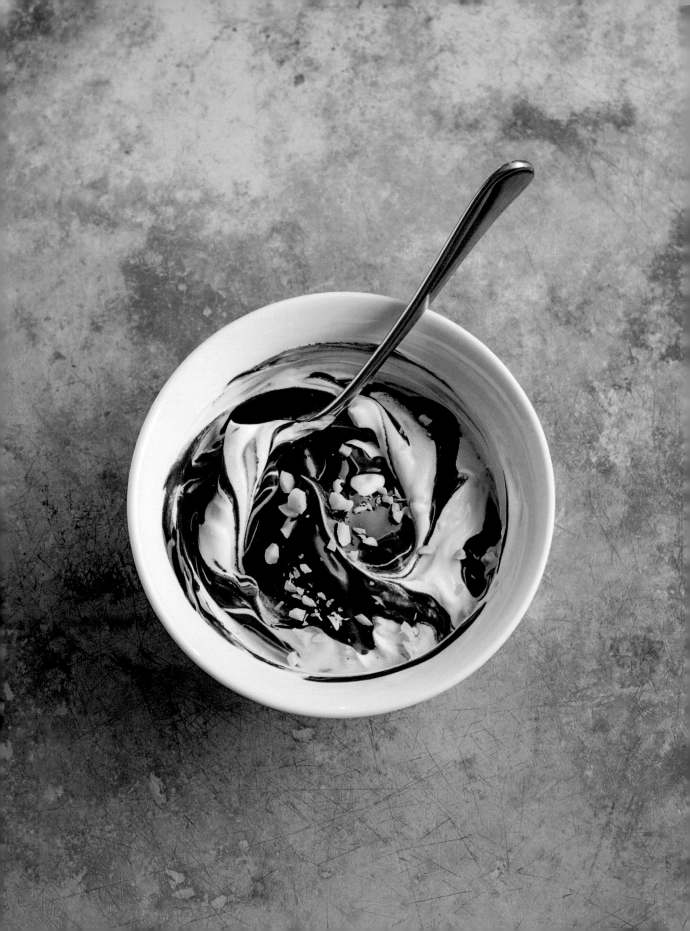

Peanut Choc Yog Pot

SERVES 1

Yoghurt pot breakfasts are a perfect alternative to cereal for those of you who wake up with a sweet tooth!

1 small pot 0% Greek
(or soy) yoghurt
(approx. 170g)
1 tbsp peanuts, chopped
sprinkle of stevia, to
sweeten (optional)
3 large squares dark
chocolate (70% or more),
roughly chopped

This recipe is easily adapted for vegans by using soy yoghurt instead of Greek yoghurt.

1. Spoon the yoghurt into a small bowl and mix in the peanuts and stevia, if using.

2. Place the chocolate and 1 tablespoon of water in a shallow microwavable cup and place in the microwave for 30 seconds, or until melted.

3. Stir the melted chocolate then pour over the yoghurt and stir again. Serve immediately or refrigerate overnight for a breakfast on the go.

FAT-LOSS

CALORIES: 387

Protein: 22g
Fats: 0.4g
Carbs: 74.3g

Eton Morning Mess

SERVES 1

A healthier, breakfast version of Eton Mess for dessert lovers!

1 small bowl (approx. 50g)
    Rice Krispies
1 small pot 0% Greek (or
    soy) yoghurt (approx.
    170g)
1 large handful
    strawberries, chopped
1 tbsp runny honey

1. Combine the Rice Krispies and yoghurt in a small bowl.

2. Add the strawberries and stir well.

3. Drizzle over the honey to serve.

This recipe is easily adapted for vegans by using soy yoghurt instead of Greek yoghurt and swapping the honey for maple syrup. You could use raspberries, blueberries or blackberries, instead of strawberries, in this dish – or you could use a combination of berries.

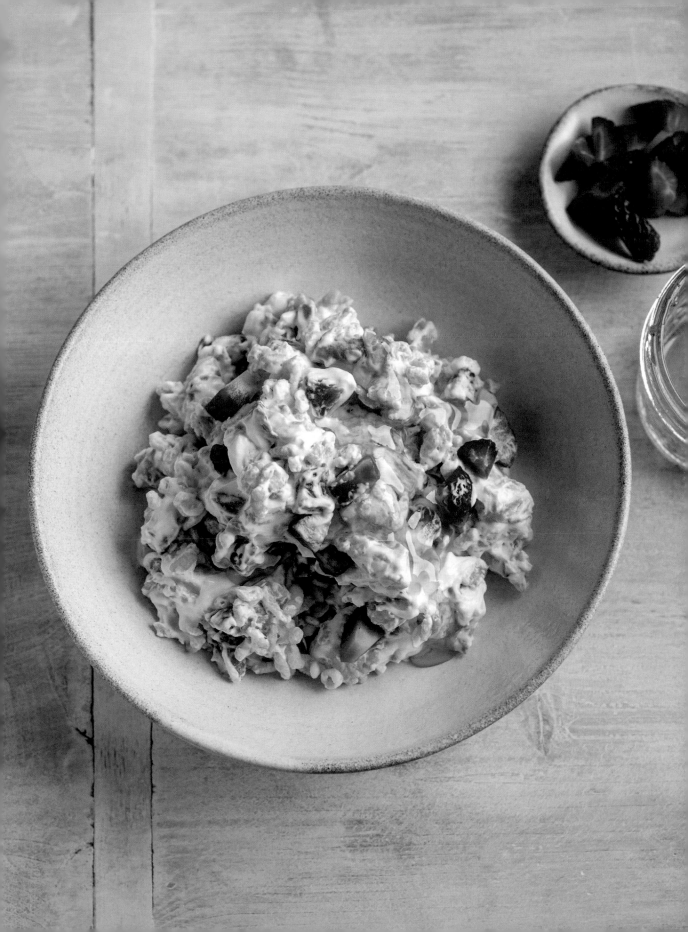

CALORIES: 395
Protein: 16.3g
Fats: 7.8g
Carbs: 68g

Spicy Overnight Oats

SERVES 1

This is my favourite breakfast when it's cold outside. Here's a new, spicy take on an old classic...

2 sachets / 2 handfuls oats
   (approx. 60g total weight)
100ml light and / or
   unsweetened soy
   milk (any)
1 small green apple, cored
   and diced or grated
4 tbsp 0% Greek (or soy)
   yoghurt
½ tsp ground cinnamon
½ tsp ground ginger
½ tsp ground nutmeg
1 tsp runny honey

1. Combine the oats and soy milk in a jar or small bowl. Add the apple and yoghurt and mix well.

2. Stir in the spices then drizzle the honey over the top.

3. Leave in the fridge for 6–24 hours before serving.

This recipe is easily adapted for vegans by using soy yoghurt instead of Greek yoghurt and swapping the honey for agave or maple syrup.

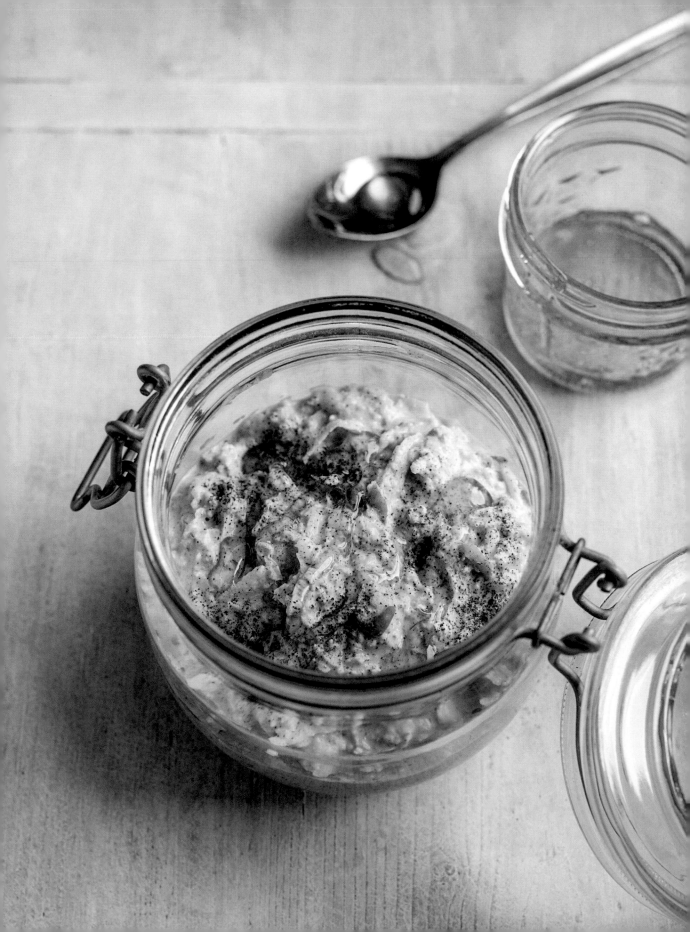

MUSCLE-BUILDING / PERFORMANCE GOALS
(high-calorie and high-macro recipes)

Hypertrophy (muscle building) is achieved with a progressive weight-lifting plan coupled with a high-calorie, high-protein and high-carbohydrate diet. These muscle-building / performance recipes are all high calorie, high protein and high carb, to help aid both your training and recovery.

Please note: Regardless of goals, I ALWAYS recommend carbohydrate consumption pre- and post-workout. If you train in the morning, I advise you to choose a higher carb recipe both before and after your training session.

MUSCLE-BUILDING
CALORIES: 674cals
Protein: 28g
Fats: 48g
Carbs: 33g

Protein Ice Cream Shake

SERVES 1

A protein shake pre- or post-workout is ideal as it's a fast-digesting, direct hit of protein. Adding some fast-release (sugary) carbs for a performance or muscle-building goal will ensure you train hard.

1 scoop protein powder
500ml unsweetened nut milk (any)
1 level tbsp crunchy nut butter
    (homemade see page 183 or
    shop-bought)
1/3 tub vanilla ice cream (approx. 150g)

1. Place all ingredients in a blender and whizz until you reach the desired consistency.

2. Pour into a glass and serve.

This recipe is easily adapted for vegans by using vegan ice cream.

MUSCLE-BUILDING
CALORIES: 625cals
Protein: 31g
Fats: 18g
Carbs: 86g

High Protein Vegan Smoothie

SERVES 1

This is a great HIGH PROTEIN breakfast smoothie for all you vegans out there!

250g soy yoghurt
1 large handful berries
1 large banana, peeled
1 sachet / 1 handful oats (approx. 30g)
500ml light and / or unsweetened soy
    or nut milk (any)

1. Place all ingredients in a blender and whizz until you reach the desired consistency.

2. Pour into a glass and serve.

MUSCLE-BUILDING

CALORIES: 672
Protein: 19g
Fats: 46g
Carbs: 53g

Bacon Avocado Toastie

SERVES 1

If you're looking for breakfast on the go, it doesn't always have to be a shake – toasties are a great breakfast to wrap in tinfoil and eat en route.

2 rashers bacon (any)
2 slices bread, wholemeal
   or sourdough (typically
   80–100g total weight)
1 tsp butter
1 small avocado, mashed
1 tsp fresh lime juice
pinch dried chilli flakes
   or dash sriracha sauce
   (optional)

This recipe is easily adapted for vegetarians by using veggie bacon.

1. Preheat the grill to high.

2. Place the bacon under the grill and cook to your preferred crispiness.

3. Meanwhile, toast and butter the bread. Spread with the mashed avocado and season with freshly ground black pepper and lime juice. Sprinkle with chilli flakes or sriracha sauce, if using.

4. Top with the bacon and serve open or as a toastie.

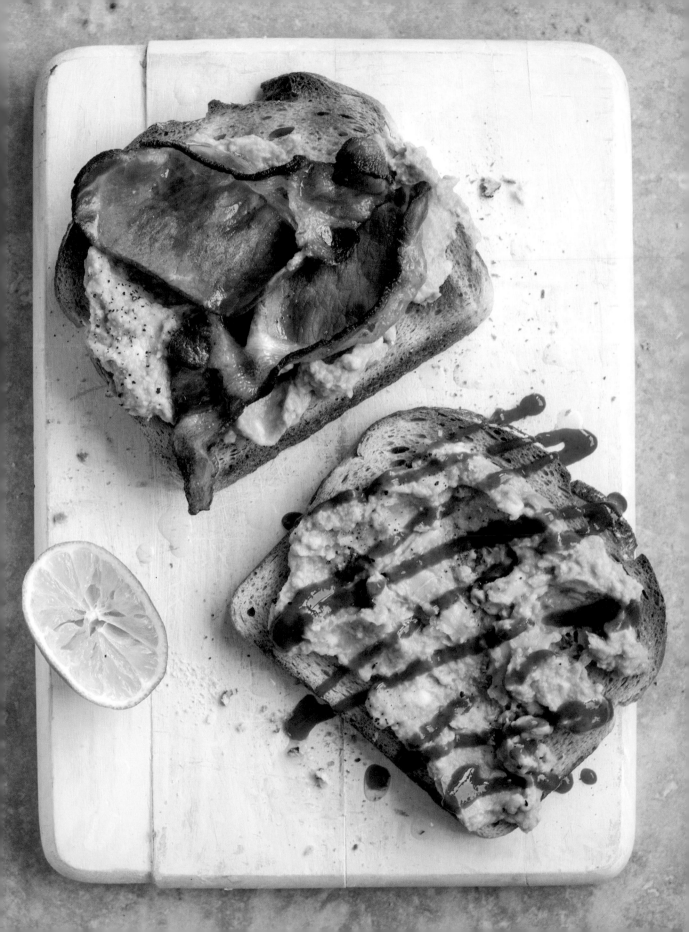

CALORIES: 524
Protein: 35g
Fats: 22g
Carbs: 44g

My New York Bagel with a Twist

SERVES 1

I feel no shame in admitting that this works best with corned beef but because I know how unpopular that is these days, I've put a healthy twist on the classic!

1 small egg
1 plain bagel
1 tsp butter
2 slices chicken or turkey
   'lunchmeat' (thinly sliced
   cooked meat)
1 slice Cheddar or any
   preferred cheese
3 slices tomato
1 lettuce leaf

This recipe is easily adapted for vegetarians by using Quorn slices instead of lunchmeat.

1. Place a non-stick frying pan over a high heat and crack the egg into the centre. Season the egg with salt and freshly ground black pepper and cook for 2–3 minutes, then flip (over easy).

2. Meanwhile, toast and butter the bagel.

3. Place the chicken or turkey on top of one half of the toasted bagel, then top with the egg, hot from the pan. Top this with the cheese (so it melts a little).

4. Finally, lay the tomato and lettuce on the meat, followed by the second half of the bagel, and serve.

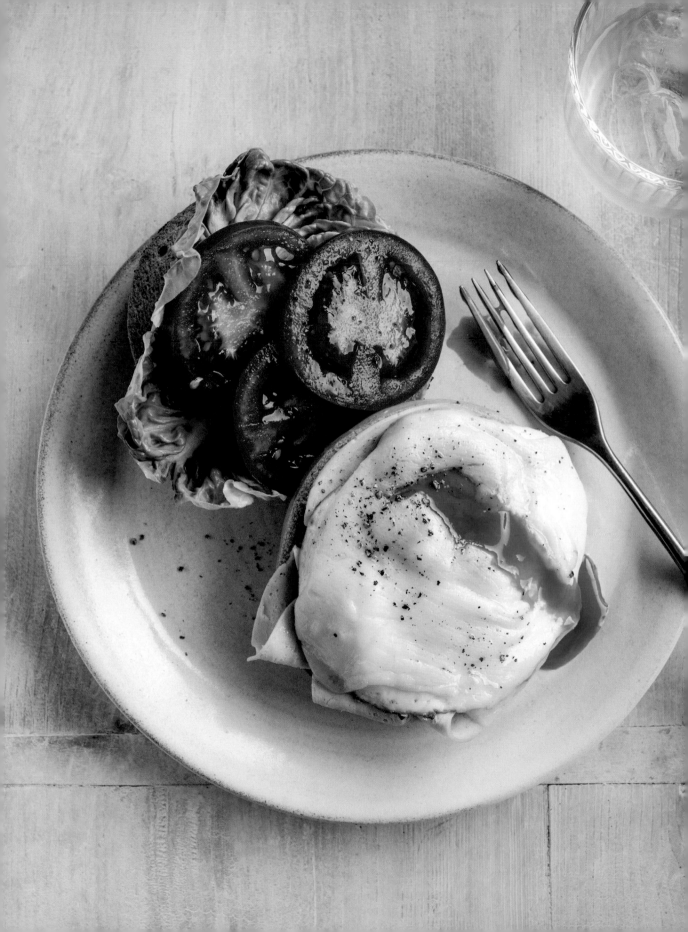

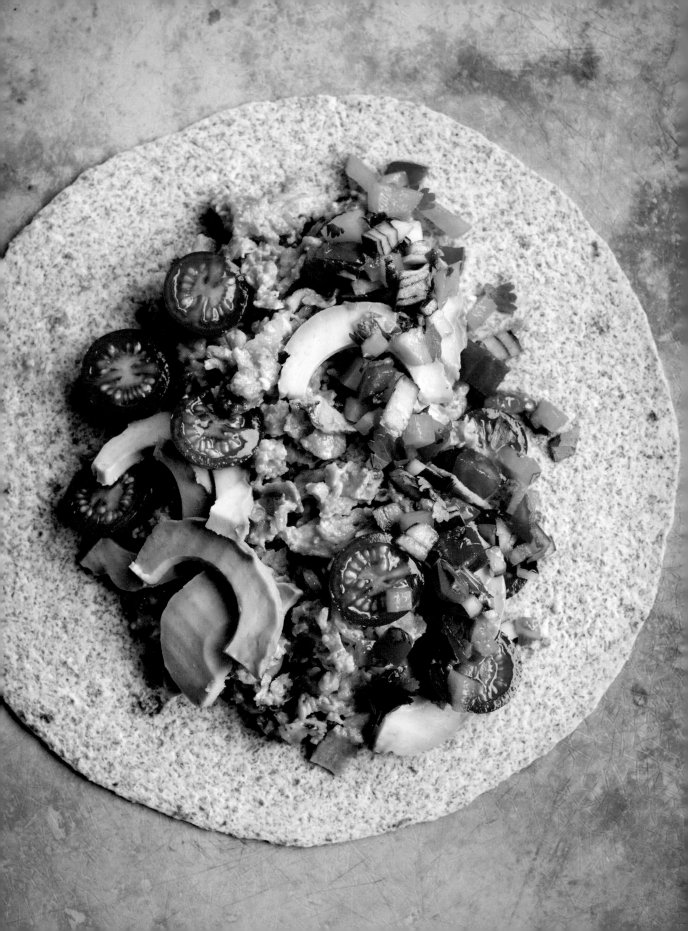

CALORIES: 547
Protein: 28g
Fats: 36g
Carbs: 31g

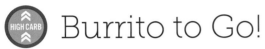

Burrito to Go!

SERVES 1

Wrapping the bottom half of your burrito in tinfoil is a great way to avoid egg drippings when you're on the go.

3 rashers bacon (any)
3 small eggs
1 large tortilla (any)
4 cherry tomatoes, halved
 or quartered
½ small avocado, sliced
1 tbsp salsa (homemade see
 page 180 or shop-bought)

1. Place a non-stick frying pan over a high heat.

2. Using a pair of scissors, chop the bacon into the hot pan.

3. When the bacon is nearing your preferred crispiness, reduce the heat to medium and crack in the eggs. Scramble everything together.

4. Meanwhile, heat the tortilla in a separate pan or in the microwave on medium (typically for 30 seconds).

5. Remove the tortilla from the heat and spoon the egg and bacon mixture into the centre. Top with the tomatoes, avocado and salsa.

6. Fold the bottom half of the tortilla over the filling and then tightly roll the wrap from right to left. Wrap in tinfoil and go!

MUSCLE-BUILDING
CALORIES: 631
Protein: 22g
Fats: 28g
Carbs: 81g

Flourless Honey Pancakes

SERVES 1

A sweet and healthy start to the day for those with a performance goal.

2 large ripe bananas
4 small eggs
1 tbsp butter
1 tbsp runny honey

COOK'S TIP

I find that small, non-stick pans are great when it comes to making foolproof pancakes and omelettes. Most supermarkets sell them, so if you have a few quid to spare, it's worth the investment.

1. Peel the bananas and mash them together in a large bowl using a fork. Don't worry if there are still a few lumps.

2. Crack the eggs into the bowl and whisk with the banana until you have a consistent texture.

3. Place the butter in a non-stick frying pan over a medium heat to melt.

4. Turn the heat up high and pour in a few dollops of the batter. As soon as the base starts to turn golden brown (this usually takes about 2–3 minutes) flip the pancakes and cook on the other side for 2–3 minutes. Remove from the heat and set aside.

5. Continue cooking until you have used all the batter (this mixture should make about 8 small or 4 large pancakes).

6. Drizzle with honey to serve.

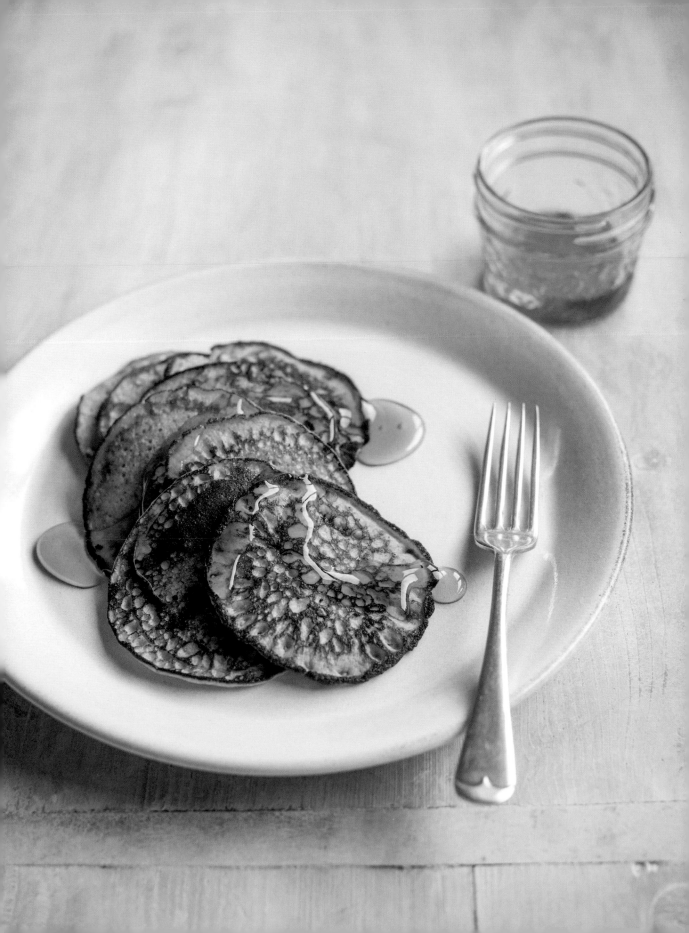

CALORIES: 500
Protein: 19g
Fats: 36g
Carbs: 27g

Tofu Scramble

SERVES 1

Lucy Watson mentioned this recipe when she was a guest on my podcast –
I tried it the following week with great success!

2 tsp olive oil
1 garlic clove, peeled
    and crushed
large pinch ground
    turmeric
2 spring onions, sliced
80g tofu
1 large handful spinach
1 large handful cherry
    or baby plum tomatoes,
    halved or quartered
1–2 basil leaves, finely
    chopped
1 large slice ciabatta bread
    (typically 40–50g)
pinch chilli flakes
    (optional)

1. Place 1 teaspoon of the oil in a non-stick frying
pan over a medium heat and add the garlic,
turmeric and spring onions. Cook for 2–3 minutes,
stirring occasionally.

2. Crumble the tofu into the pan and cook for
2–3 minutes.

3. Stir in the spinach and tomatoes and season
with salt and freshly ground black pepper. Cook
for a further 2–3 minutes, then add the basil.

4. Meanwhile, toast or griddle the ciabatta and
brush with the remaining oil.

5. Top the toast with the tofu scramble, sprinkle
with the chilli flakes, if using, check the seasoning
and serve.

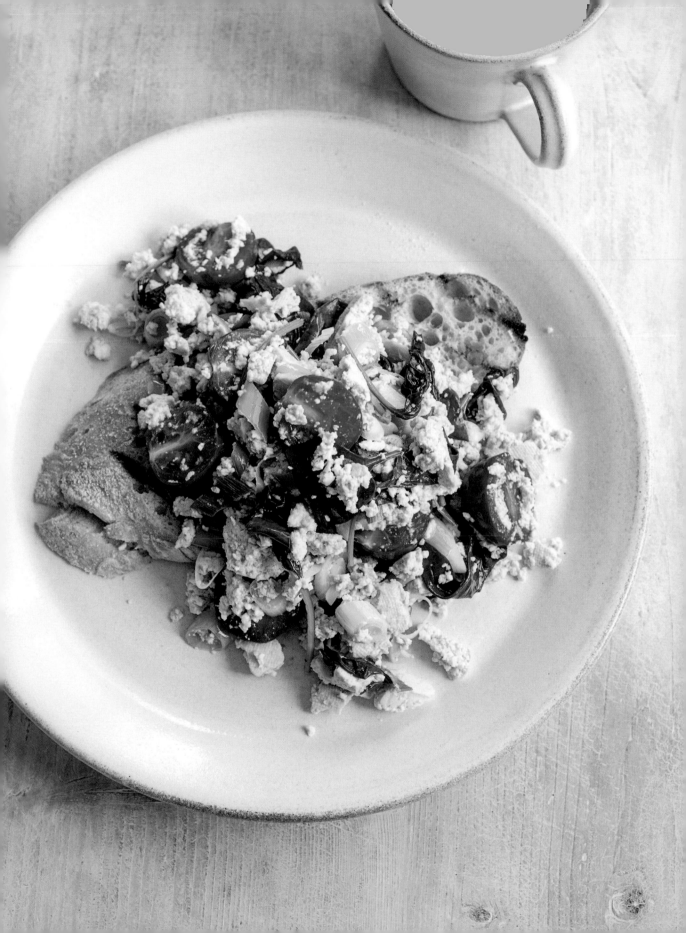

CALORIES: 704
Protein: 35g
Fats: 39g
Carbs: 55g

American Toast

SERVES 1

If you have a muscle-building goal, it's important that your meals are high in both protein AND carbohydrates, allowing you to train effectively and recover optimally. Adding slow-release carbs or simple sugars to your morning protein will do the trick nicely.

1 tsp butter
4 rashers bacon (any)
3 small eggs
½ tsp ground cinnamon (optional)
2 large slices bread (typically 80–100g total weight)
1 tbsp maple syrup (any)

This recipe is easily adaptable for vegetarians simply by using veggie bacon instead of bacon.

1. Place the butter in a large non-stick frying pan over a medium heat to melt.

2. Swirl the pan to coat in the melted butter then add the bacon. Fry to your desired crispiness, then remove from the pan and set aside.

3. Meanwhile, whisk the eggs in a large bowl and season with either cinnamon (to make sweet toast) or salt and freshly ground black pepper (to make them savoury). Lay the first piece of bread in the egg mixture and gently push it down with your fingertips to coat. Remove to a side plate then repeat the process with the second slice.

4. Lay both pieces of bread in the pan and turn the heat up to high. After 2–3 minutes, when the base is golden brown, flip the toast to fry on the other side. After a further 2–3 minutes, remove them from the pan and place on a plate.

5. Top with the bacon and drizzle with the syrup to serve.

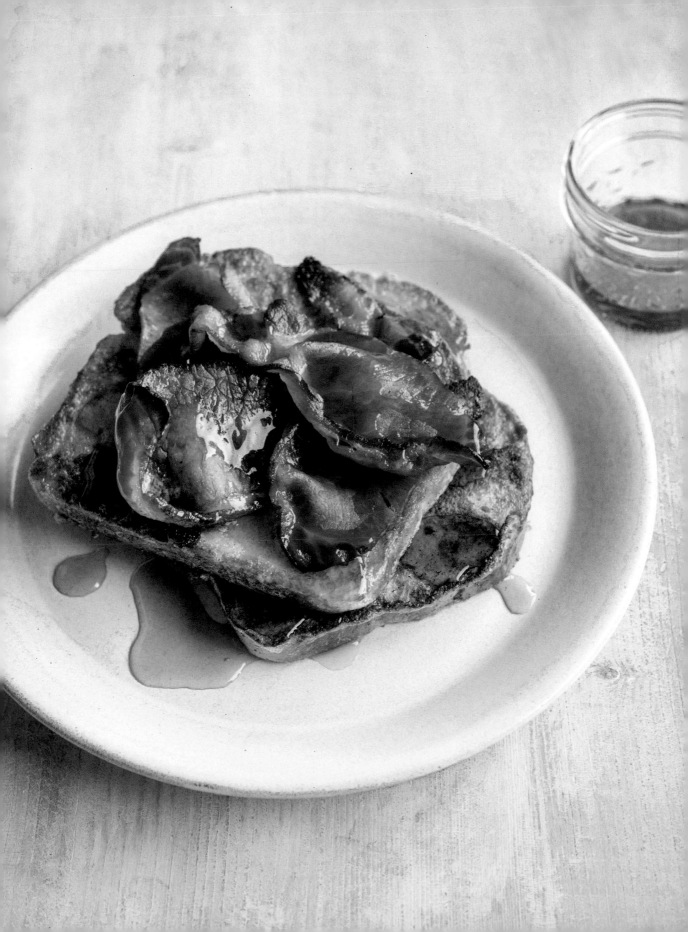

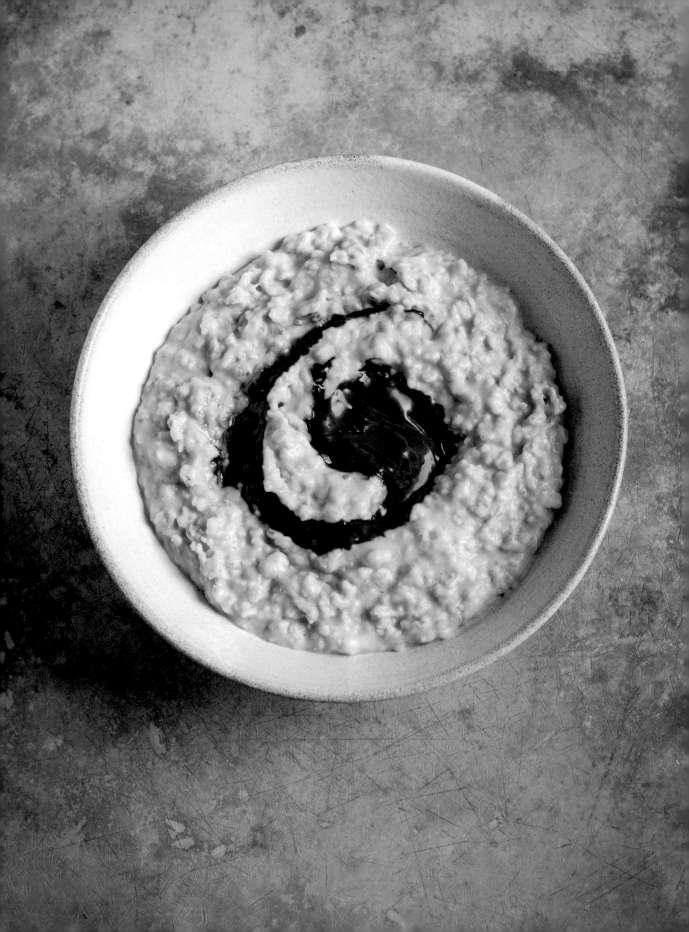

Melt-in-the-Middle Protein Oats

SERVES 1

This is a great breakfast for on-the-go lifters. It could also be a goal-focused 'treat' on a cold day!

1 sachet / 1 handful oats (approx. 30g)
1 scoop protein powder
approx. 300ml unsweetened nut milk (any)
2 tbsp Nutella (or other preferred spread)

1. Mix the oats, protein powder and milk together in a bowl and microwave for 2 minutes on a high heat.

2. Remove the bowl from the microwave and spoon one dollop of Nutella, immediately followed by the second, into the centre of the porridge. Place back in the microwave for a further 30 seconds.

3. Remove and serve.

This recipe is easily adapted for vegans by using a vegan spread instead of Nutella.

MUSCLE-BUILDING

CALORIES: 735
Protein: 25g
Fats: 36g
Carbs: 75g

Chocolate Chip Granola Pot

SERVES 1

A high-carb, high-protein, portable pot that's perfect for a pre- or post-workout feed.

2 large squares dark
   chocolate (the darker
   the better), chopped
   into pieces
250ml 0% Greek (or soy)
   yoghurt
100g granola
   (homemade see page 184
   or shop-bought)
1 tsp nut butter
   (homemade see page 183
   or shop-bought)

1. Using a bowl or large jam jar, stir the chocolate pieces into the yoghurt.

2. Mix in the granola and spoon the nut butter over the top.

3. Cover the bowl or place a lid on the jam jar and refrigerate overnight, or simply eat and go!

This recipe is easily adapted for vegans by using soy yoghurt instead of Greek yoghurt and choosing vegan chocolate and vegan granola.

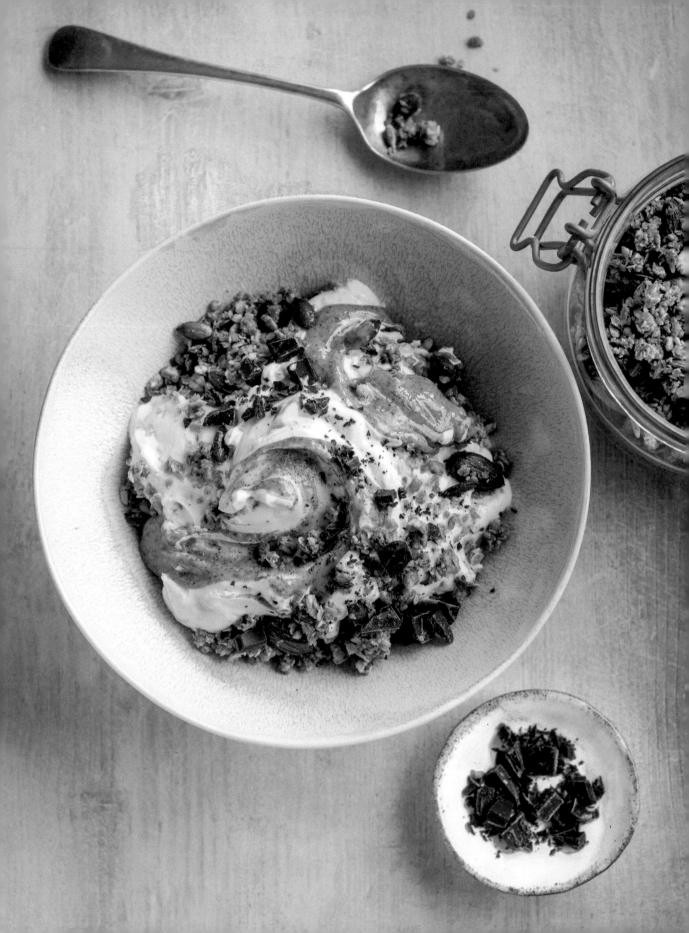

GENERAL HEALTH AND FITNESS GOALS

(well-balanced calorie and macro recipes)

General health and fitness goals should have a happy dietary balance of calories and macronutrients, which is exactly what I have tried to cater to in these recipes.

*Please note: Regardless of goals, I ALWAYS recommend carbohydrate consumption pre- and post-workout. If you train in the morning, I advise you to choose a higher carb recipe both before and after your training session. If you train fasted, that's fine, just make sure to have a higher carb recipe **post** training.*

CALORIES: 471
Protein: 14g
Fats: 24g
Carbs: 48g

Good Gut Grains

SERVES 1

High fibre cereal = good gut health
Dark chocolate = antioxidant
Peanut butter = a complete protein when combined with a wholegrain
This is a FANTASTICALLY healthy breakfast!

2 large handfuls All-Bran
    cereal (approx. 60g)
approx. 300ml
    unsweetened nut milk
    (any)
pinch of stevia, to sweeten
    (optional)
2 squares dark chocolate
    (the darker the better),
    broken into small pieces
1 level tbsp crunchy nut
    butter (homemade see
    page 183 or shop-bought)

1. Place the All-Bran in a small bowl, cover with the milk and sprinkle in the stevia, if using.

2. Stir the chocolate into the cereal and spoon in the nut butter. Microwave on high for approximately 1 minute, allowing the chocolate to melt a little and the nut butter to soften.

3. Remove from the microwave, stir and serve!

GENERAL HEALTH

CALORIES: 423
Protein: 24g
Fats: 21g
Carbs: 34g

Breakfast Pizzette

SERVES 1

A hearty, healthy breakfast pizza.

1 wholewheat tortilla
⅓ tin chopped tomatoes
   (approx. 130g)
½ red onion, peeled and
   finely sliced into rings
1 large handful spinach
1 large handful rocket
½ block halloumi, sliced
   then torn
1 large egg
4 fresh basil leaves

1. Preheat the grill to medium.

2. Place the tortilla on a baking tray and spoon the chopped tomatoes over the top in a circular motion so they reach the outer edge of the wrap.

3. Sprinkle with the onion rings, then scatter the spinach and rocket over the top. Season everything well with salt and freshly ground black pepper. Arrange the halloumi over the green leaves then place under the grill for 5–10 minutes, until the halloumi is golden brown (it won't melt much) and the tortilla edges are crispy.

4. Meanwhile, place a small frying pan over a medium heat. Crack in the egg and cook to your preference.

5. Remove the pizzette from the grill, top with the egg, scatter over the basil, season with freshly ground black pepper and serve.

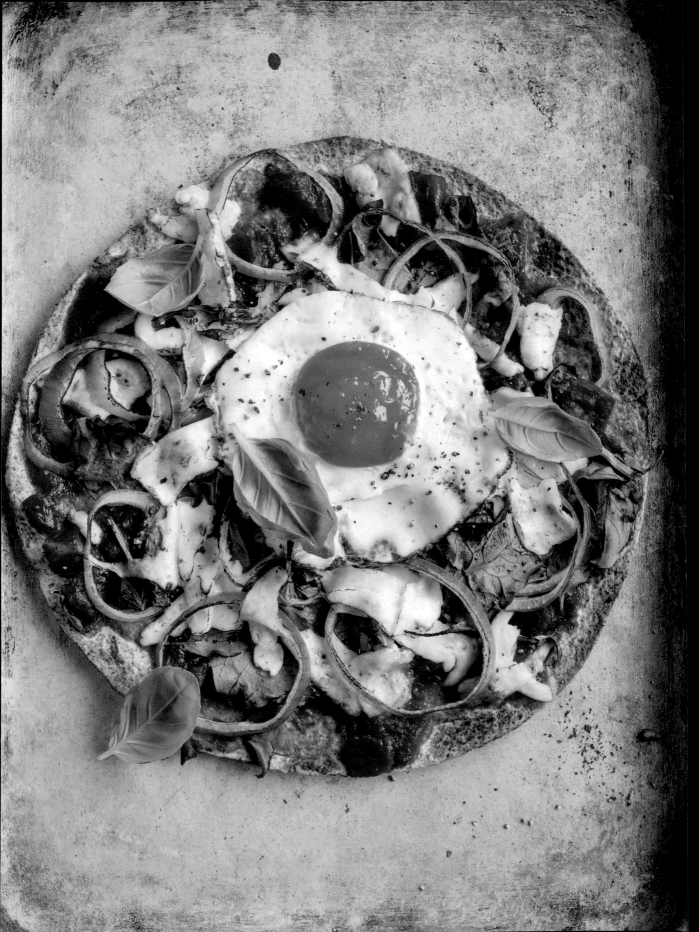

CALORIES: 461
Protein: 23.9g
Fats: 23.6g
Carbs: 38.6g

Mushroom and Potato Frittata

SERVES 1

If you don't have a frying pan small enough then combine all the ingredients in an oven dish and cook for 20–25 minutes in an oven preheated to 190°C/ Fan 170°C. Serve this frittata with a green salad.

1 tbsp butter
1 large handful mushrooms
    (any), halved or sliced
300g cooked new potatoes,
    sliced
3 large eggs
handful fresh parsley,
    roughly chopped

You could leave the potatoes out of this frittata and serve it with a hunk of sourdough instead.

1. Melt the butter in a large ovenproof frying pan over a medium heat.

2. Add the mushrooms and season well with salt and freshly ground black pepper. Cook for 6–7 minutes until they are starting to brown, then add the potatoes. Stir to mix well.

3. Whisk the eggs in a small bowl and stir in the parsley. Pour the eggs into the pan and turn the heat down low. Cook for 8–10 minutes until almost set.

4. Meanwhile, preheat the grill to medium-high.

5. When the frittata is almost set, place under the grill to cook for 3–5 minutes, until golden brown on top.

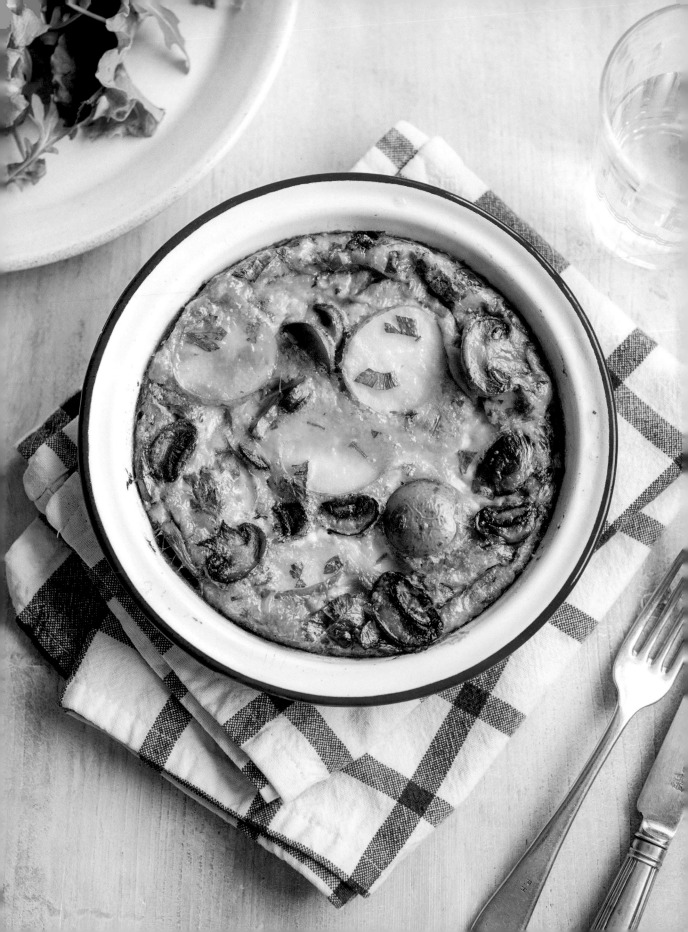

GENERAL HEALTH

CALORIES: 476
Protein: 19g
Fats: 28g
Carbs: 37g

Poached Eggs and Avocado on Toast

SERVES 1

If it ain't broke...

½ large avocado, mashed
pinch dried chilli flakes
   or paprika (optional)
squeeze lime juice
1 tbsp vinegar
2 small eggs
2 slices wholemeal bread
   (typically 80–100g
   total weight)
1 tsp butter

1. Place the avocado in a small bowl and season with chilli or paprika, if using, and a squeeze of lime juice. Mix well.

2. Bring a saucepan of water to the boil and reduce it to a gentle simmer. Add the vinegar and swirl the water with a spoon into a mini cyclone. Crack one egg gently into the centre of the swirling water, swiftly followed by the second. Cook the eggs for approximately 2–3 minutes.

3. Meanwhile, toast and butter the bread, then spread with the avocado.

4. Remove the eggs from the pan with a slotted spoon, then slide gently on top of the toast. Season with salt and freshly ground black pepper and serve.

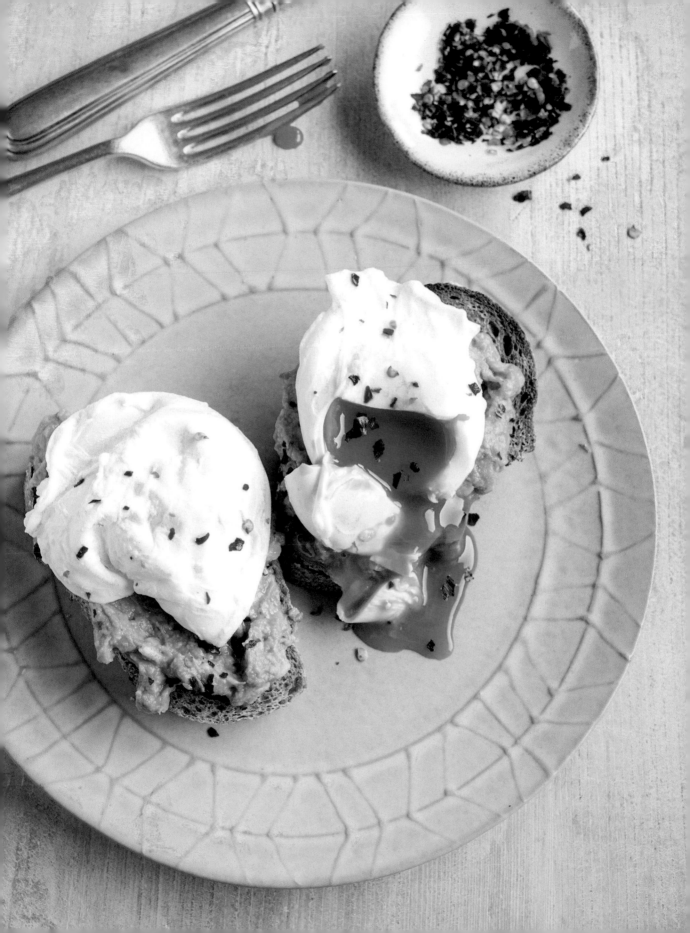

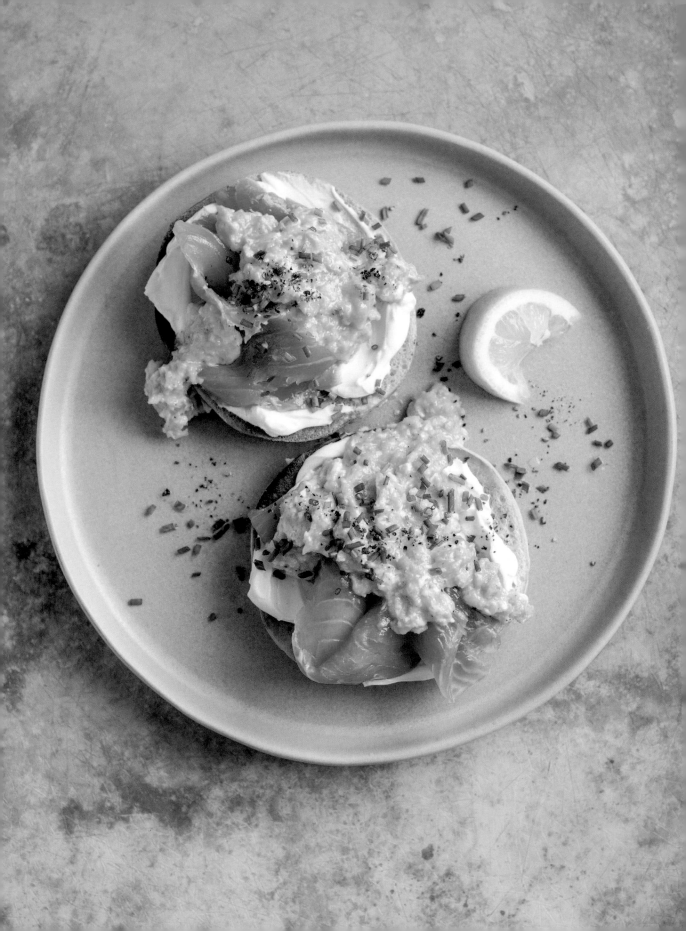

Smoked Salmon Scramble

SERVES 1

Salmon is one of the best dietary fats you're going to find, as are eggs, and BOTH double up as a complete protein source. These two macronutrients are essential for your physical health and wellbeing... This is also one of the tastiest breakfasts in the world!

1 bagel thin
2 level tbsp cream cheese
½ small packet smoked salmon (approx. 50g), roughly chopped with scissors
1 tsp butter
2 small eggs
1 tbsp chopped fresh chives (optional)
lemon wedge, to serve (optional)

1. Toast the bagel and spread with the cream cheese. Top with the smoked salmon.

2. Meanwhile, melt the butter in a non-stick frying pan over a medium heat.

3. Crack the eggs into the pan, season with salt and freshly ground black pepper, and start to scramble with a wooden spoon.

4. When the eggs are cooked to your desired consistency, spoon on to the bagel, sprinkle with the chives, if using, and serve.

COOK'S TIP

Bagel thins are great for keeping foods that you love in your diet when you are being a bit calorically minded. I'd rather my readers reduce carbs than fats, as fats are the more nutritional of the two macros.

The Nutrient Omelette

SERVES 1

This is a really yummy omelette FILLED with nutritious ingredients! Feel free to serve up with a side of breakfast veg, such as mushrooms, tomatoes and spinach.

1 tsp butter
1 large handful kale
1 small handful pine nuts
3 small eggs
1 small handful goat's
    cheese, crumbled

1. Melt the butter in a non-stick frying pan over a medium heat, then chuck in the kale and pine nuts.

2. When the kale has wilted and the pine nuts are slightly toasted, remove from the pan and set aside

3. Crack the eggs into a small bowl, season well with salt and freshly ground black pepper and whisk. Pour the egg mixture into the pan and swirl in a circular motion so it spreads and cooks evenly. Use a spatula to pull in the sides of the omelette to allow any uncooked mixture to reach the surface of the pan.

4. Top the wet omelette with the kale and pine nuts, followed by the goat's cheese, and continue to cook.

5. When the omelette has cooked to your preferred consistency (I like mine a little runny, but it's up to you), fold over and slide on to a plate to serve.

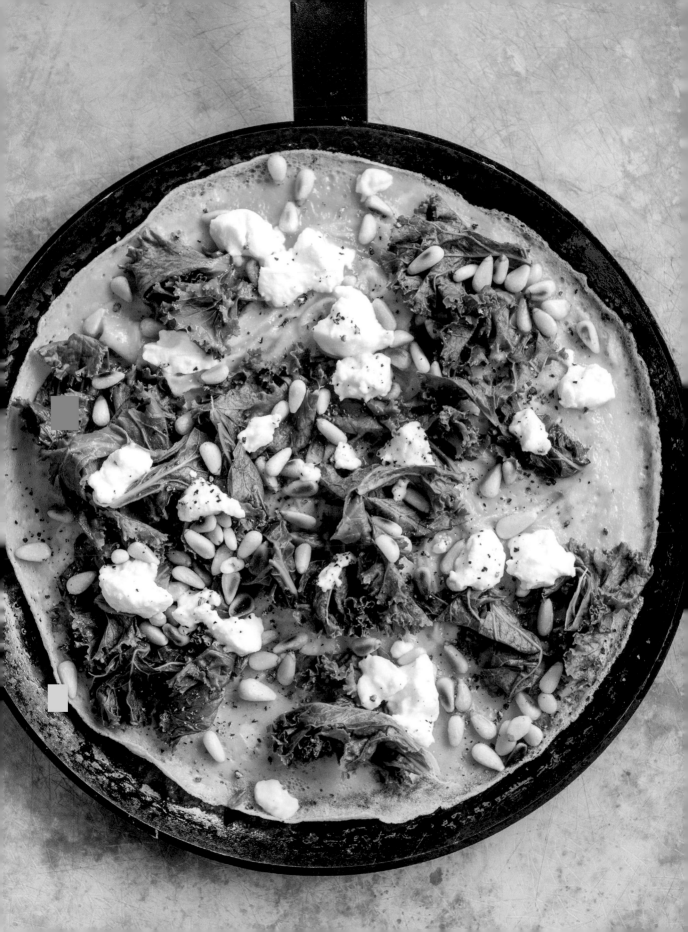

GENERAL HEALTH

CALORIES: 455
Protein: 45g
Fats: 12g
Carbs: 45g

Blueberry Protein Pancakes

SERVES 1

This is a super-healthy breakfast of berries, proteins and fats – perfect for a health-conscious goal.

2 scoops protein powder
2 small eggs
dash unsweetened nut
   milk (any)
1 large handful blueberries,
   halved
1 tbsp honey

1. Whisk the protein powder with the eggs in a small bowl to make a thick batter. Depending on the protein powder you use, you may need to add up to 100ml milk. Only add the milk in small dashes, though, until you reach the desired consistency. Stir in the blueberries.

2. Place a non-stick frying pan over a high heat and pour in your first portion of pancake batter. As soon as the pancake forms edges (this should take about 1 minute), turn the heat down to medium and leave to cook for 1–2 minutes, until brown.

3. Flip the pancake over and cook for a further 1–2 minutes. Remove from the pan and set aside.

4. Repeat this process until all the batter is used up.

5. Stack the pancakes on a plate, drizzle over the honey and serve!

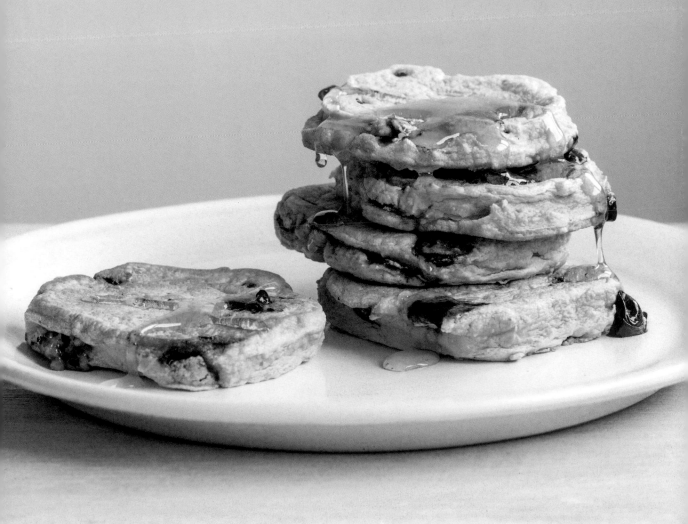

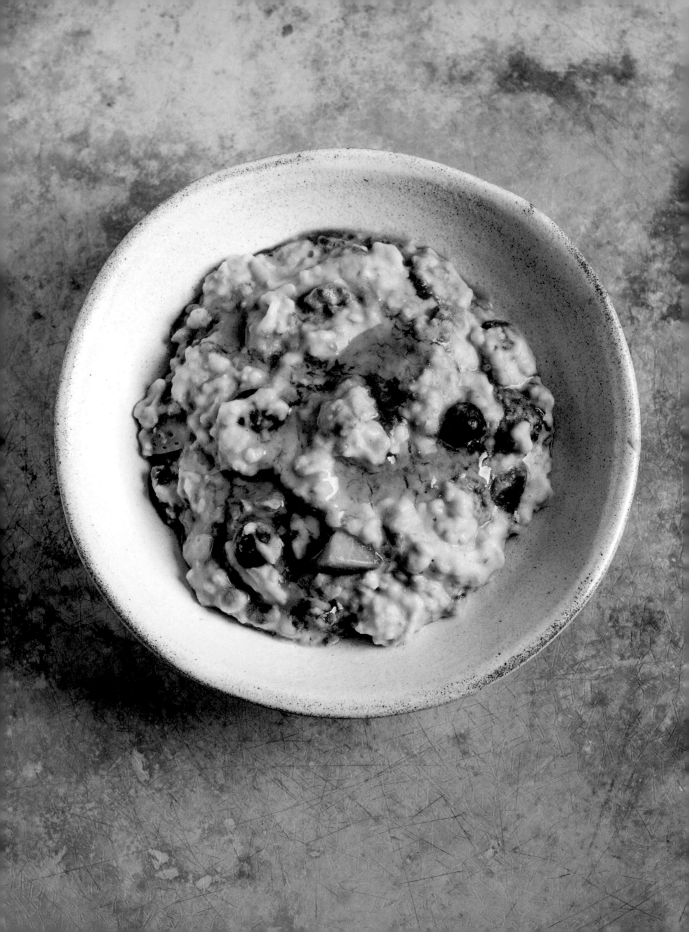

Antioxidant Protein Porridge

SERVES 1

This is a super-healthy, super-macro-friendly recipe.

1 sachet / 1 handful oats
(approx. 30g)
1 scoop protein powder
approx. 300ml
unsweetened nut milk
(any)
1 large handful mixed
berries
1 tbsp maple syrup

1. Combine the oats, protein powder and milk in a large bowl and stir well.

2. Microwave on high for 2 minutes.

3. Remove the bowl from the microwave and stir well. Add the berries and return to the microwave for a further 2 minutes. (You can add the berries at the end if you'd prefer, but I like it when they ooze into the oats a little!)

4. Remove the porridge from the microwave, drizzle or stir in the maple syrup and serve.

GENERAL HEALTH

CALORIES: 489
Protein: 15g
Fats: 15g
Carbs: 76g

Vit C Smoothie

SERVES 1

I don't recommend 'juicing' all day but morning, pre- and post-workout shakes are a great way to get your calories in and save on time!

1 small orange, peeled and diced
1 small apple, cored and diced
1 small handful strawberries
250ml soy yoghurt
approx. 500ml light and / or
    unsweetened soy milk
1 large handful ice (optional)

1. Place all ingredients in a blender and whizz until you reach the desired consistency.

2. Pour into a glass and serve.

GENERAL HEALTH

CALORIES: 517
Protein: 12g
Fats: 16g
Carbs: 83g

The Matcha Smoothie

SERVES 1

I'm wary of using buzz words because they often give the wrong impression, but let's just say that matcha, fruit, wholegrains and nuts are probably one of the most nutrient dense combinations you will find. This is a great smoothie for all my health-conscious readers.

1 tsp matcha powder (any)
1 small green apple, peeled, cored and
    roughly chopped
1 small pear, peeled, cored and roughly
    chopped
1 handful spinach
1 small banana, peeled
1 sachet / 1 handful oats (approx. 30g)
1 level tbsp nut butter (homemade see page
    183 or shop-bought)
approx. 300ml unsweetened nut milk (any)

1. Place all ingredients in a blender and whizz until you reach the desired consistency.

2. Pour into a glass and serve.

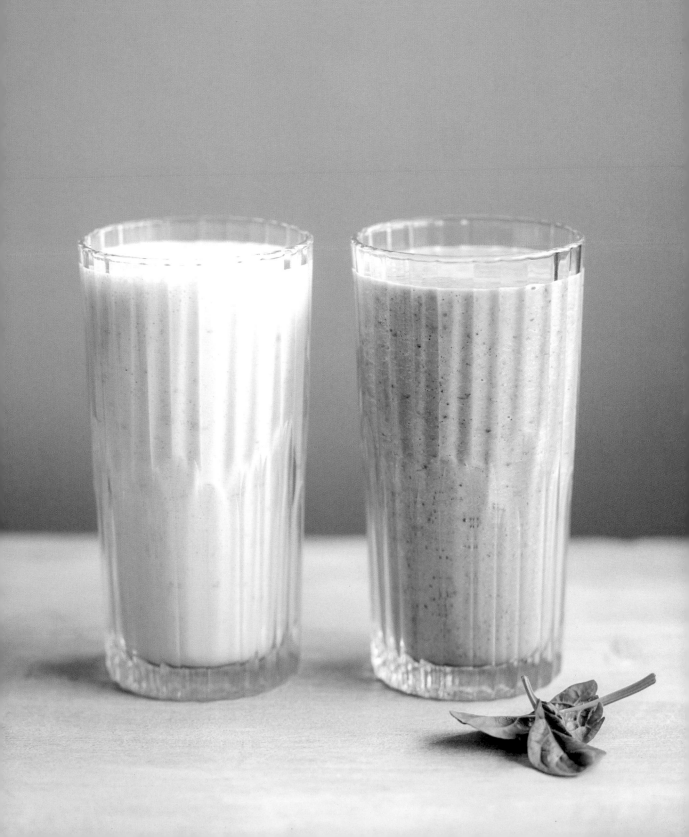

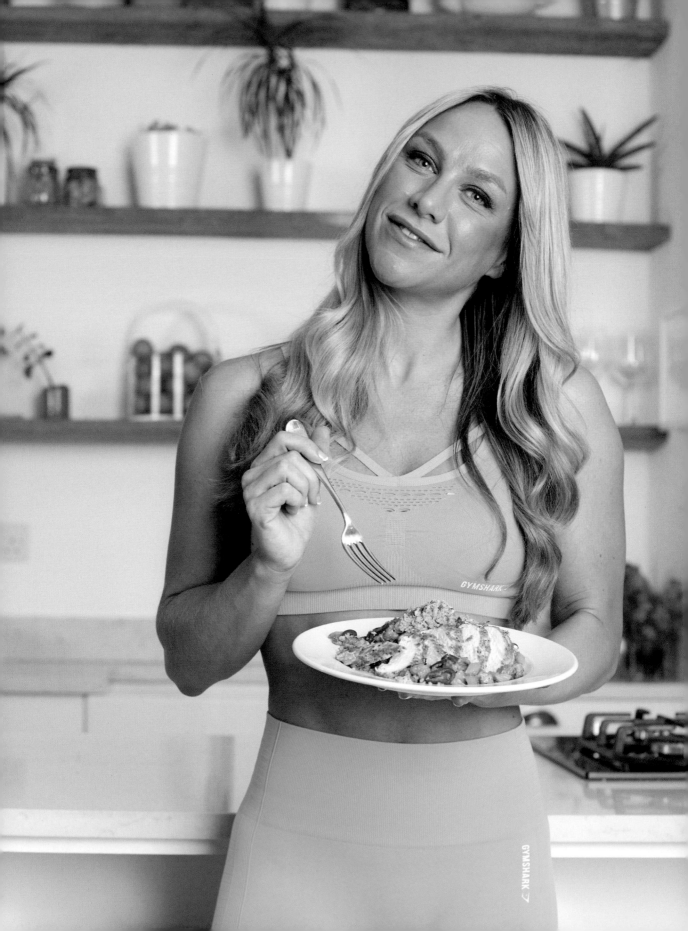

LUNCH
AND
DINNER

● ● ●

My clients will often use my recipes as
calorie- and macro-appropriate meal ideas,
while making the recipes their own. If you'd
rather use fish than chicken, for example,
rice instead of pasta, or avocado instead
of oil, feel free to do this, switching up
your various macronutrient sources.

FAT-LOSS GOALS
(low-calorie and high-protein recipes)

Fat loss is only achieved when you are in a calorie **deficit** (the number of calories you consume via food needs to be smaller than the number of calories you use via movement; this is called a Negative Energy Balance).

These fat-loss recipes are ALL low in calories and high in protein, with different quantities of the two energy macros (fats and carbs), according to your preference.

Please note: Regardless of goals, I ALWAYS recommend carbohydrate consumption pre- and post-workout.
If your lunch or dinner is pre- or post-workout, I advise you choose a higher carb recipe both before and after your session.

Fast Fried Rice

SERVES 1

Healthy protein, fats and carbs, this is a great macro dish!

1 tsp sesame oil
1 tsp chopped, crushed
   or puréed garlic
1 tsp chopped or
   puréed chilli
½ tsp ground cinnamon
   (ideally not 'sweet'
   cinnamon – the darker,
   spicier kind)
½ packet microwave brown
   rice (approx. 125g)
2 small eggs
1 large handful peas
   (frozen or fresh)
1 tsp light soy sauce
1 spring onion,
   roughly chopped

1. Place the sesame oil in a wok or large non-stick frying pan over a high heat. Add the garlic, chilli and cinnamon. When the oil starts to spit, add the rice and toss everything together. Cook for 2–3 minutes.

2. Break the eggs directly into the wok and mix together with a wooden spoon so the eggs scramble into the rice. Add the peas and soy sauce and continue to toss for a further 1–2 minutes.

3. Tip the fried rice into a bowl and sprinkle the spring onion over the top to serve. Season with a dash more soy, if desired.

This recipe is easily adapted for vegans by using tofu instead of eggs.

FAT-LOSS

CALORIES: 389
Protein: 17.6g
Fats: 15.5g
Carbs: 42g

The Healthy PB & J

SERVES 1

The wholemeal and nut butter combine to make this a complete protein sarnie. Add the fruit and you have yourself a sweet and indulgent yet VERY healthy lunch!

2 slices wholemeal bread (typically 80–100g total weight)
2 level tbsp crunchy peanut butter (homemade see page 183 or shop-bought)
6 large strawberries, sliced

1. Smear the slices of bread with the peanut butter.

2. Place the strawberries evenly over the peanut butter. Sandwich the bread together and serve.

You can have this toasted, if you like (my husband prefers it this way), but traditionally the bread should be soft.

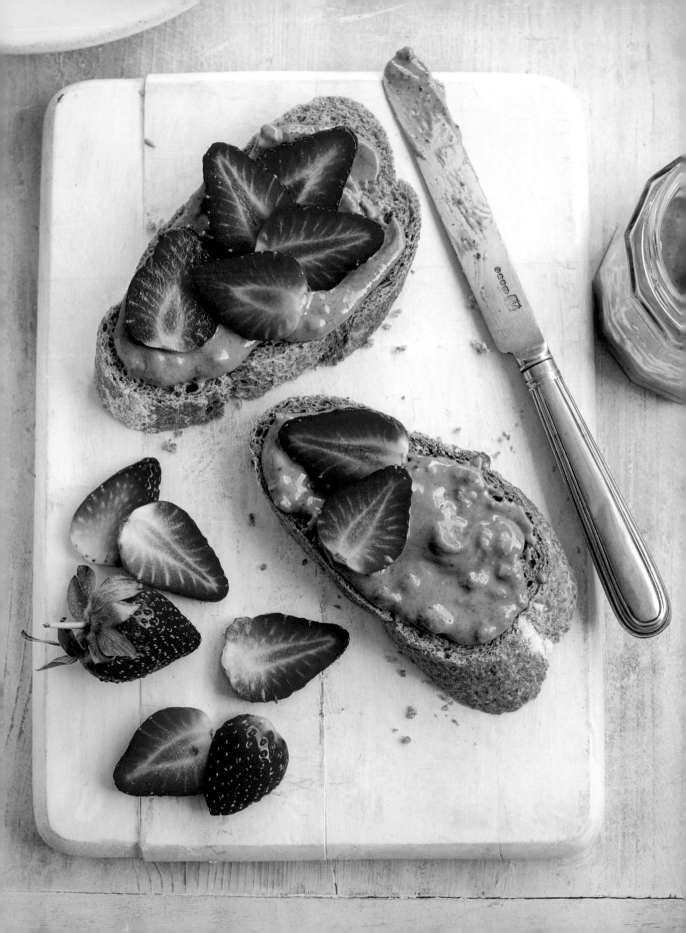

FAT-LOSS

CALORIES: 398
Protein: 16.9g
Fats: 2.6g
Carbs: 70.9g

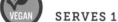

Mexican Bean and Brown Rice Bowl

SERVES 1

The beans and rice make a complete protein so this is a great high-carb, high-protein, low-fat meal for anyone who trains. The calories are LOW so don't be scared of the carbs – it's the calories that count, remember!

2 small handfuls (approx. 60g) brown rice (approx. 125g cooked weight)
½ tsp ground turmeric (optional)
½ small red onion, peeled and roughly chopped
1 tsp chopped, crushed or puréed garlic
1 small red chilli, chopped
½ × 400g tin chopped tomatoes
½ × 400g tin red kidney beans, drained
1 jalapeño pepper, sliced
pinch paprika (optional)
1 handful fresh coriander, roughly chopped, to serve (optional)

COOK'S TIP

If you are in a hurry, use ½ packet microwavable brown rice instead.

1. Place the rice in a saucepan with the turmeric and cook according to the packet instructions.

2. Meanwhile, place the red onion in a non-stick saucepan over a medium-high heat and cook for 3–5 minutes to soften. Add the chopped garlic and chilli and cook for a further minute.

3. Add the tomatoes and bring to a simmer.

4. Add the kidney beans and half the jalapeño pepper, season with salt, freshly ground pepper and paprika, if using, then mix well.

5. Once the rice is cooked, drain if necessary, then add to the pan and continue to simmer for a further 1–2 minutes.

6. Tip into a bowl, sprinkle with the remaining jalapeño and the fresh coriander, if using, to serve.

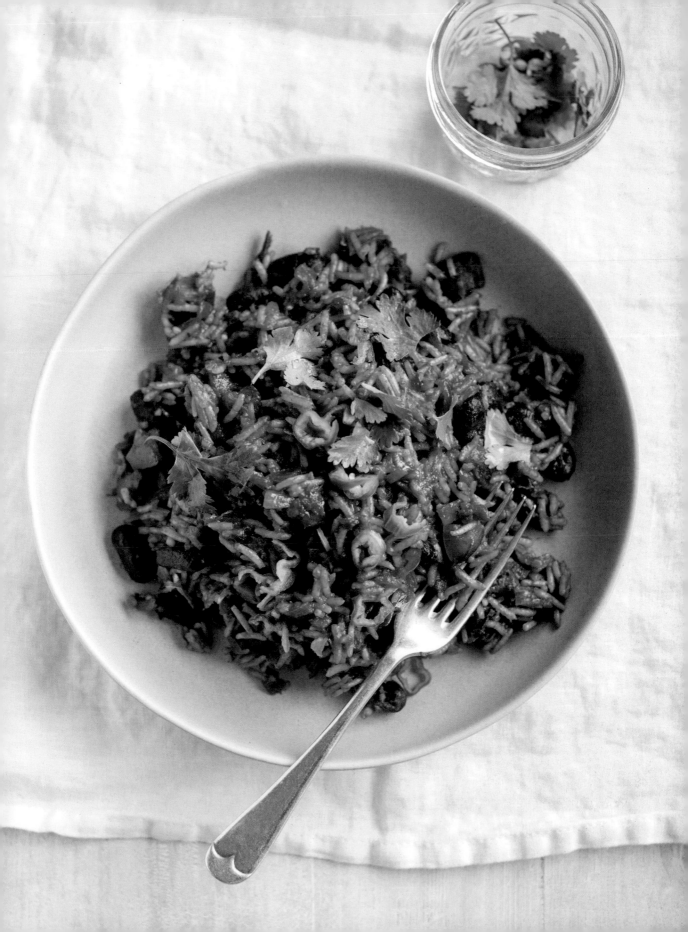

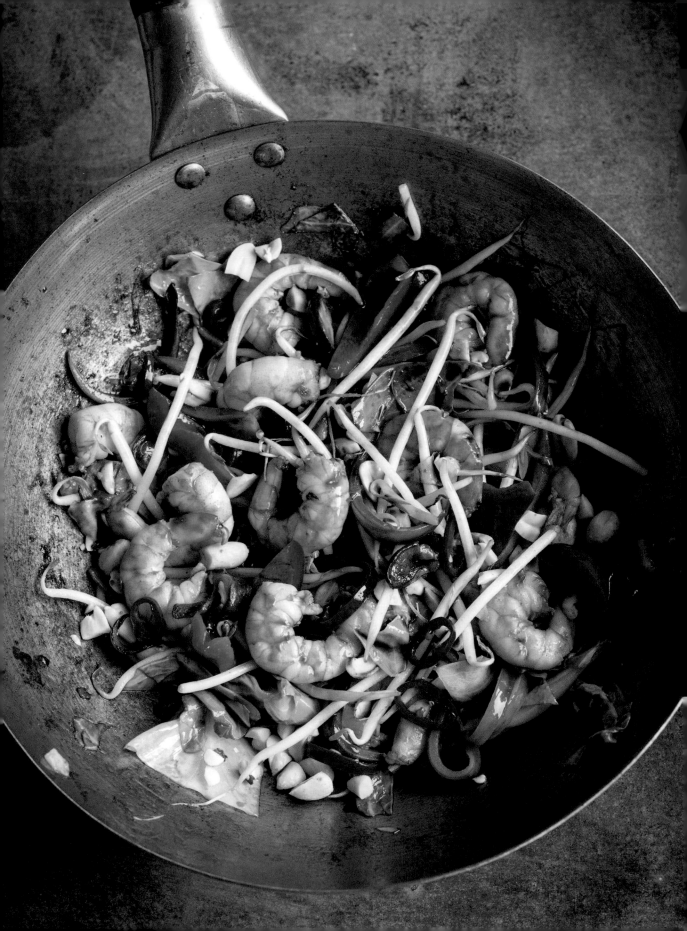

Prawns, Shoots and Leaves

SERVES 1

High protein, high fibre, high health!

1 tbsp sesame oil
1 chilli, diced
1 tsp chopped, crushed
   or puréed garlic
1 small packet raw prawns
   (approx. 150g)
1 large handful mushrooms
   (I like shiitake but any
   will do), sliced
1 large handful beansprouts
½ small red onion, peeled
   and sliced
½ small red pepper,
   chopped
1 large handful green
   cabbage, chopped
1 tbsp light soy sauce
1 small handful peanuts
   or cashews, roughly
   chopped

1. Place the sesame oil in a wok or large non-stick frying pan over a high heat. When the oil starts to spit, add the chilli and garlic to the pan.

2. Throw in the prawns and toss them with the chilli and garlic until they start to turn pink.

3. Add all the veg and cook for 3–4 minutes (I like my stir fries super crunchy but if you like softer veg, cook it for longer).

4. Add the soy sauce and continue to toss.

5. Tip the contents into a bowl, sprinkle over the nuts and serve.

This recipe is easily adapted for vegans and vegetarians by using tofu instead of prawns. If you are in a hurry, use 150g ready-prepared stir-fry veg (approx. ½ packet).

FAT-LOSS

CALORIES: 360
Protein: 23.4g
Fats: 14g
Carbs: 36.3g

Smoked Salmon Wraps

SERVES 1

Salmon is one of the best sources of fats in the world. When you see it on a menu or find it at the supermarket, grab it!

2 small tortilla wraps
2 level tbsp light cream
   cheese
2 thick slices smoked
   salmon (approx. 40g)
juice of ½ lemon
2 large handfuls
   salad leaves

1. You can have the tortillas soft and eat this cold (my mum likes it that way), but I prefer to warm the wraps gently in a dry frying pan or griddle for 30–60 seconds on each side.

2. Spread a tablespoon of cream cheese on each of the wraps.

3. Top with the salmon and season with freshly ground black pepper.

4. Squeeze over the lemon juice and place a large handful of the salad leaves in the middle of each wrap. I like to use rocket.

5. Tuck the bottom of the wrap under, then tightly roll each wrap from left to right to serve.

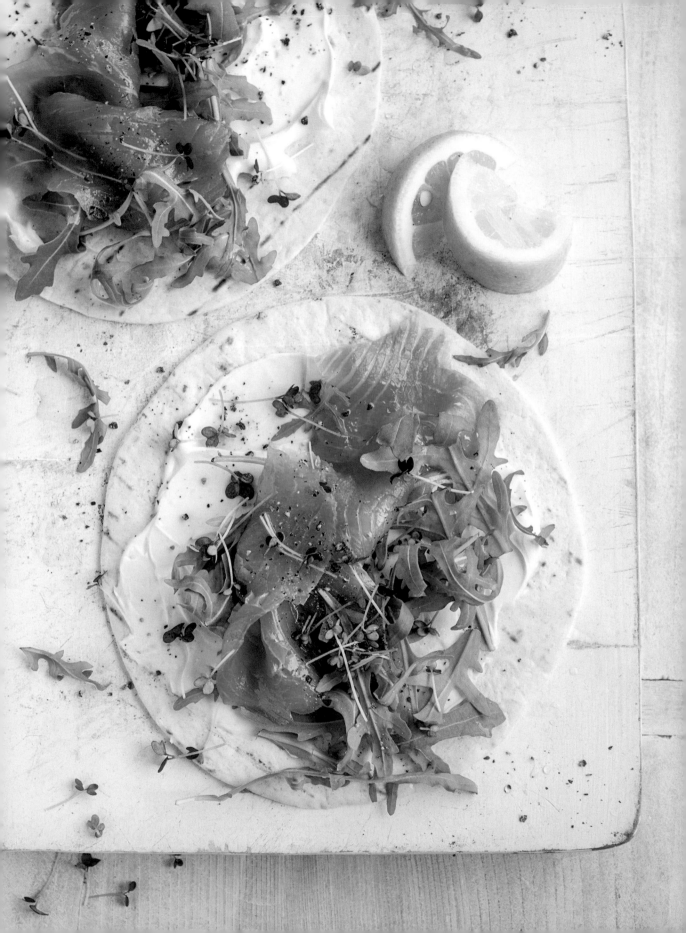

FAT-LOSS

CALORIES: 421
Protein: 38g
Fats: 11g
Carbs: 37g

Fish, Chips and Crunchy Sprouts!

SERVES 1

A healthier, crunchier take on the original of this recipe, which is in my first book, *The 4-Week Body Blitz*.

3 large new potatoes,
   quartered lengthways
1 large handful baby
   sprouts, trimmed
   and halved
1 small cod fillet
   (typically 120g)
1 small egg, beaten
1 sachet / 1 handful oats
   (approx. 30g)
1 tbsp reduced salt and
   sugar ketchup (optional)

The calorie and macro quantities for the potatoes are 90cals, 2g protein, 20g carbs and no fat, so if you want to serve the fish without the extra carbs then do!

1. Preheat the oven to 200°C/Fan 180°C.

2. Bring a small saucepan of salted water to the boil. Add the potatoes and boil for 10 minutes. Add the sprouts to the pan and cook with the potatoes for 5 minutes.

3. Drain the potatoes and sprouts and lay them out on a large baking tray before seasoning well with salt and freshly ground black pepper (I like using garlic salt, too). Bake in the oven for 10 minutes.

4. Meanwhile, dip the fish in the beaten egg, coating it evenly.

5. Add the oats to a separate bowl, then place the fish in the oats and make sure to cover it evenly.

6. Remove the tray from the oven and add the fish. Season well and bake for 15 minutes until golden brown.

7. Plate up with the ketchup, if using, and serve.

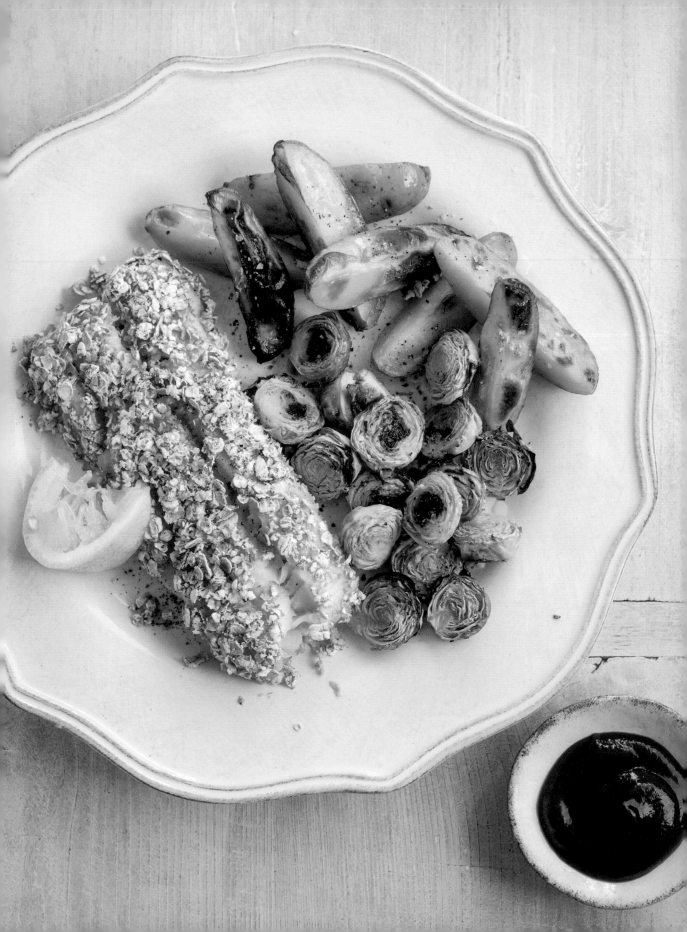

CALORIES: 366
Protein: 38.5g
Fats: 15.3g
Carbs: 20.2g

Traybake Salmon and Fennel

SERVES 1

My editors suggested we have a few more traybake recipes in the book, as they are super quick and easy. If you can throw some protein, veg and whatever else into a tray and bake it, then do!

½ onion (any), peeled and
  cut into thin wedges
1 fennel bulb, sliced
50g new potatoes, halved
1 tsp olive oil
1 fillet salmon
  (typically 120g)
½ lemon
1 handful fresh parsley,
  roughly chopped

This recipe is easily adapted for vegetarians and vegans by using Quorn or tofu instead of salmon.

1. Preheat the oven to 200°C/Fan 180°C.

2. Place the onion, fennel and potatoes on a baking tray and drizzle with the oil. Season with salt and freshly ground black pepper and cook in the oven for 10–15 minutes.

3. Remove the tray from the oven and turn the potatoes and fennel. Place the salmon fillet on top of the veg and squeeze the lemon over the fish. Cut the squeezed lemon shell in half and add to the tray with the veg. Season the fish well and return the tray to the oven for 10–15 minutes, until the salmon is cooked through and the veg are golden.

4. Scatter over the parsley and serve.

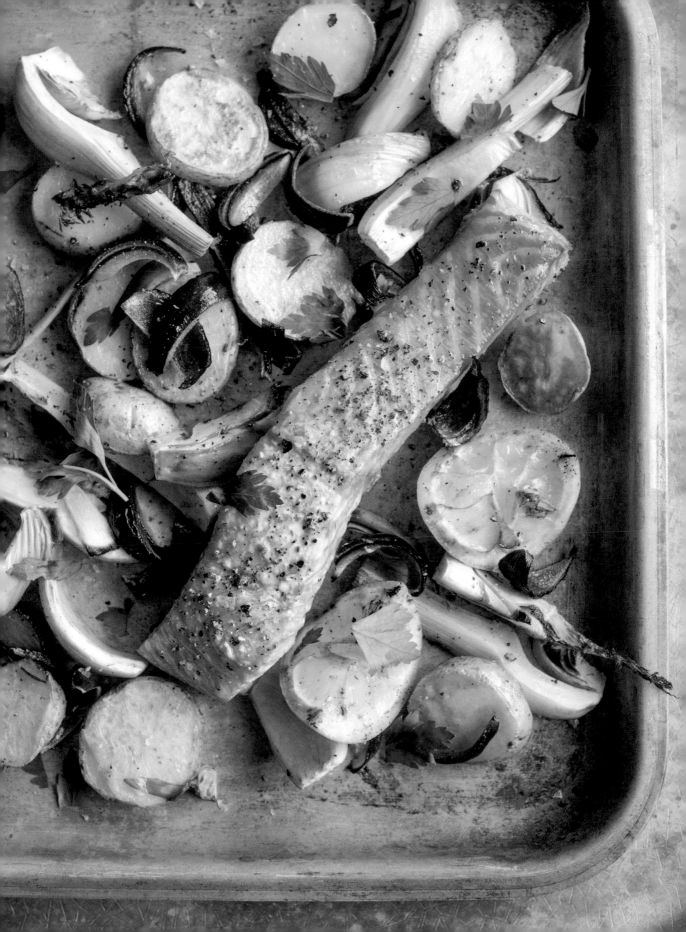

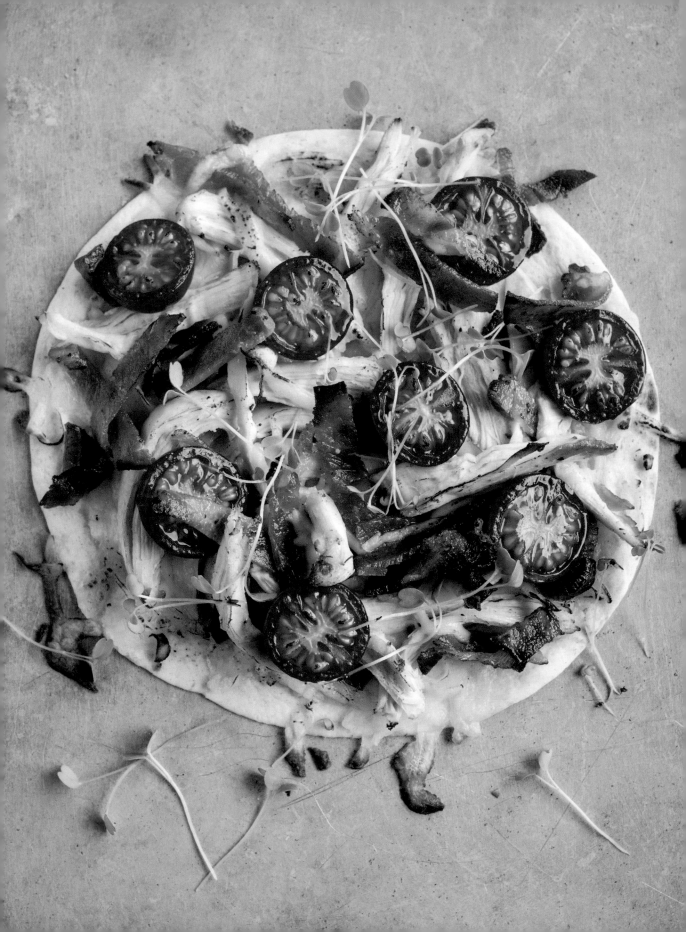

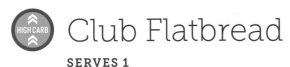

Club Flatbread

SERVES 1

A calorie-friendly take on a club sandwich.

1 small tortilla wrap
1 small handful grated
   mozzarella
1 cooked chicken breast
   (typically 125–150g),
   torn into strips
3 rashers crispy cooked
   bacon, roughly chopped
4 cherry tomatoes, halved
   or quartered
1 handful cress (optional)

1. Preheat the grill to medium.

2. Place the flatbread on a tray and sprinkle the mozzarella over the top. Add the strips of chicken. Scatter the bacon over or in between the chicken strips, then top with the tomatoes. Place under the grill for 2–3 minutes.

3. Remove from the grill, season with salt and freshly ground black pepper, sprinkle with cress, if using, and serve.

FAT-LOSS

CALORIES: 326
Protein: 45.9g
Fats: 11.7g
Carbs: 9.5g

Torn Mozzarella and Chicken Salad

SERVES 1

Feel free to bulk up your salad with more leafy greens and all of your favourite non-starchy veg. I like adding salad leaves, tomatoes, cucumbers, onions, mushrooms and peppers.

1 chicken breast
  (typically 125–150g)
1 large bowl leafy greens,
  rinsed
1 large handful cherry
  tomatoes, quartered
2 handfuls mozzarella, torn
1 tbsp balsamic vinegar
4–5 fresh basil leaves, torn

This recipe is easily adapted for vegetarians by replacing the chicken with a Quorn fillet or two hard-boiled eggs.

1. Preheat the oven to 200°C/Fan 180°C.

2. Season the chicken breast well with salt and freshly ground black pepper and cook in the oven for 15–20 minutes, until the juices run clear.

3. Remove the chicken from the oven and leave to cool for 10 minutes.

4. Meanwhile, place the salad leaves in a large bowl and add the tomatoes and mozzarella.

5. Slice the chicken into strips and scatter over the salad.

6. Dress with the balsamic vinegar and basil leaves and serve.

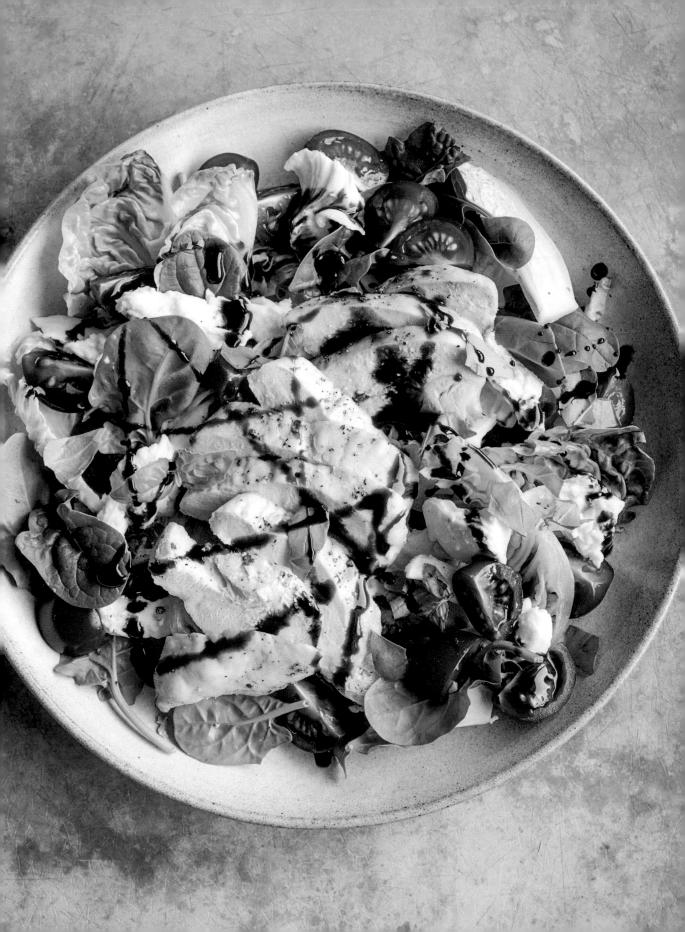

FAT-LOSS

CALORIES: 335
Protein: 44.8g
Fats: 12.3g
Carbs: 14.1g

Curried Chicken and Broccoli Rice

SERVES 1

My husband makes this chicken dish for me all the time. It's one of the only things he can cook but it's absolutely delicious!

1 tbsp curry powder
4 heaped tbsp 0% Greek
　(or soy) yoghurt
1 chicken breast or Quorn
　fillet (typically 125–150g)
1 large head broccoli or
　packet pre-riced broccoli
1 large handful chopped
　or whole almonds
1 tsp mustard seeds
½ red chilli, sliced
　(optional)
lemon wedges, to serve
　(optional)

This recipe is easily adapted for vegetarians by choosing a Quorn fillet instead of chicken.

COOK'S TIP

If you don't have any mustard seeds, then use another tablespoon of curry powder in the broccoli instead.

1. Preheat the oven to 180°C/Fan 160°C.

2. Mix the curry powder in a bowl with the Greek yoghurt then coat the chicken in the mixture.

3. Make a small bed out of tinfoil and place the chicken and any left-over marinade inside. Cook for 20–30 minutes, until the juices run clear.

4. Meanwhile, rice the broccoli using a ricer or chop finely and finish it off in a blender (I find it easier to buy pre-riced broccoli from the supermarket but you don't need to do this). Place the broccoli in a bowl and microwave on high for 2–3 minutes.

5. Place a dry frying pan over a high heat and add the almonds and mustard seeds. When the nuts start to brown and the seeds start to pop remove from the heat. Stir the toasted almonds and mustard seeds into the cooked broccoli.

6. Remove the chicken from the oven, cut into slices and season with salt and freshly ground black pepper. Serve with the almond broccoli rice, topped with chilli slices, if using, and lemon wedges alongside.

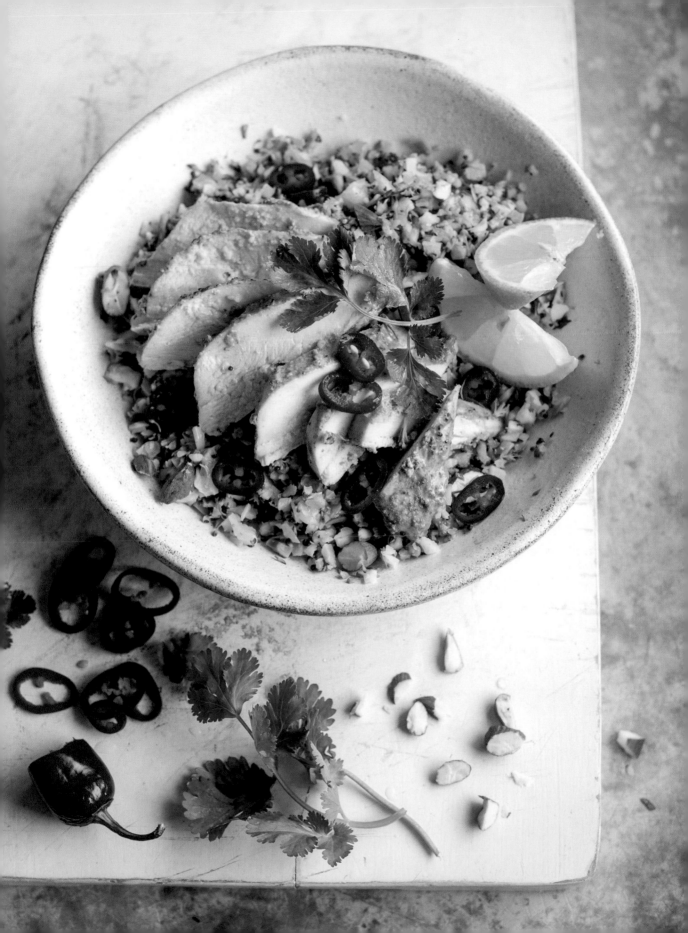

FAT-LOSS

CALORIES: 323
Protein: 47.2g
Fats: 20.5g
Carbs: 3.4g

Fillet Steak and Mushroom Medley

SERVES 1

Low carb, low calorie and yet VERY filling. This is one of those meals that will come to your rescue when dieting!

1 small fillet steak
   (typically 200g)
2 tsp salted butter
1 large garlic clove, peeled
   and chopped, crushed
   or puréed
1 large handful mixed
   mushrooms, halved or
   sliced depending on size
1 large bag spinach
1 tbsp reduced salt and
   sugar ketchup (optional)

1. Make sure the steak has been sitting at room temperature for an hour before cooking.

2. Place a frying pan over a high heat and add 1 teaspoon of the butter.

3. When the pan is hot, place the steak in the middle and sear it quickly on both sides. Once seared, leave the steak to cook for 2–6 minutes on each side, depending on your preference (2 for rare, 4 for medium rare and 6 minutes for well done).

4. Remove the steak from the pan and leave to rest while you cook the veg.

5. Return the pan to the heat with the steak juices and add the remaining butter and the garlic to the pan. Stir in the mushrooms, season well with salt and freshly ground black pepper and toss for 3–4 minutes.

6. Add the spinach and continue to toss for a further 2–3 minutes.

7. Remove the veg from the heat and serve with the steak (which you can now season), and the ketchup, if using.

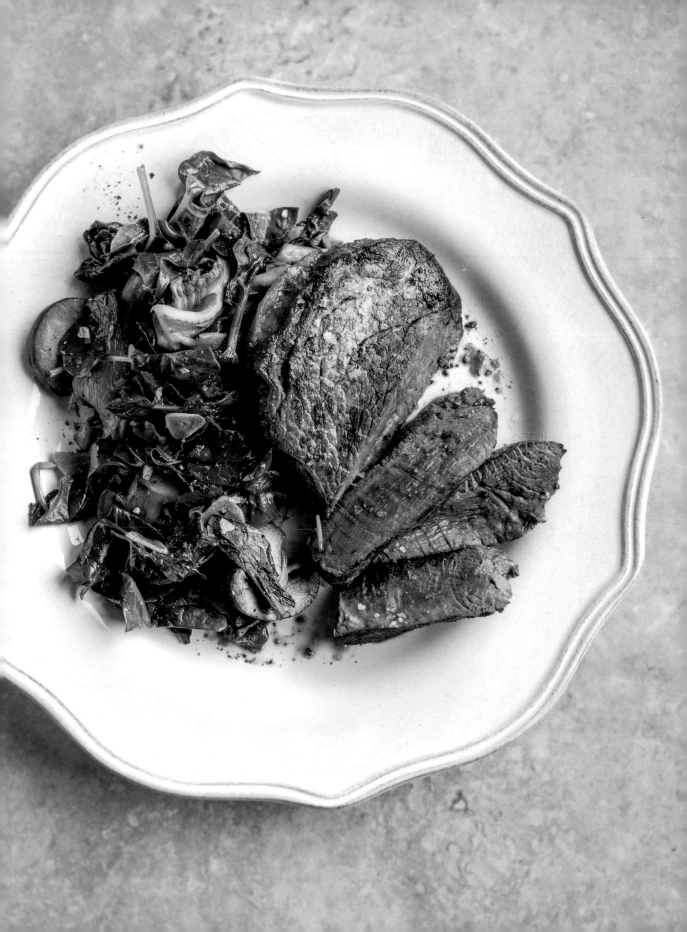

MUSCLE-BUILDING /
PERFORMANCE GOALS
(high-calorie and high-macro recipes)

Hypertrophy (muscle building) is achieved with a
progressive weight-lifting plan coupled with a high-calorie,
high-protein and high-carbohydrate diet. These muscle
building / performance recipes are all high calorie, high
protein and high carb, to help aid both your training
and recovery.

*Please note: Regardless of goals, I ALWAYS recommend
carbohydrate consumption pre- and post-workout.
If your lunch or dinner is pre- or post-workout, I advise
you choose a higher carb recipe both before and after
your session.*

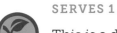

Tofu Hummus Wraps

SERVES 1

This is a double hit of protein – both the tofu AND the combination of chickpeas and wholegrains are complete proteins!

2 wholewheat tortillas
4 heaped tbsp hummus
(any)
½ packet tofu pieces
(typically 80g)
1 tomato, thinly sliced
1 large handful lettuce
(any green leaves)

1. Warm the wraps in the microwave on high for 30 seconds, or in a dry frying pan over a high heat for 30 seconds on each side.

2. Remove the wraps from the heat and spoon 2 tablespoons of hummus into the centre of each one, then spread the hummus out evenly over the wraps.

3. Place the tofu pieces in a bowl and warm in the microwave for a few minutes, or place them in a non-stick frying pan over a medium heat to warm; otherwise, serve them cold.

4. Divide the tofu, tomato slices and lettuce evenly between the wraps, scattering them into the centre.

5. Fold up the bottom of each wrap, then roll tightly from one end to the other.

CALORIES: 722
Protein: 29g
Fats: 33g
Carbs: 82g

High Protein Quesadilla

SERVES 1

A vegan quesadilla with a protein hit!

½ red pepper, thinly sliced
½ red onion, peeled and
    thinly sliced
½ packet tofu pieces
    (approx. 80g)
pinch chilli powder, garlic
    salt and / or smoked
    paprika (optional)
2 wholewheat tortillas
6 slices vegan cheese
    (or approx. 90g grated)

COOK'S TIP

You can turn this vegan quesadilla into a meat feast by swapping the tofu for cooked chicken and using Cheddar instead of vegan cheese.

1. Place the pepper, onion and tofu in a non-stick frying pan over a medium heat and cook for 4–5 minutes.

2. Once the veg and tofu have softened, place them in a bowl and set aside. Sprinkle with chilli powder, garlic salt and smoked paprika, if using.

3. Wipe the inside of the pan with some kitchen roll then return to the heat. Place one tortilla flat inside it, then place 3 slices of cheese on top of it.

4. Scatter the pepper, onion and tofu over the cheese slices then lay the remaining cheese slices on top. Finish with the second tortilla.

5. Cook for 3–4 minutes on one side, then place the flat of your hand on top of the quesadilla and push down gently, to compact it. Use a spatula and your hand to flip the quesadilla over and cook it for a further 3–4 minutes on the other side.

6. Remove from the heat, cut into wedges and serve!

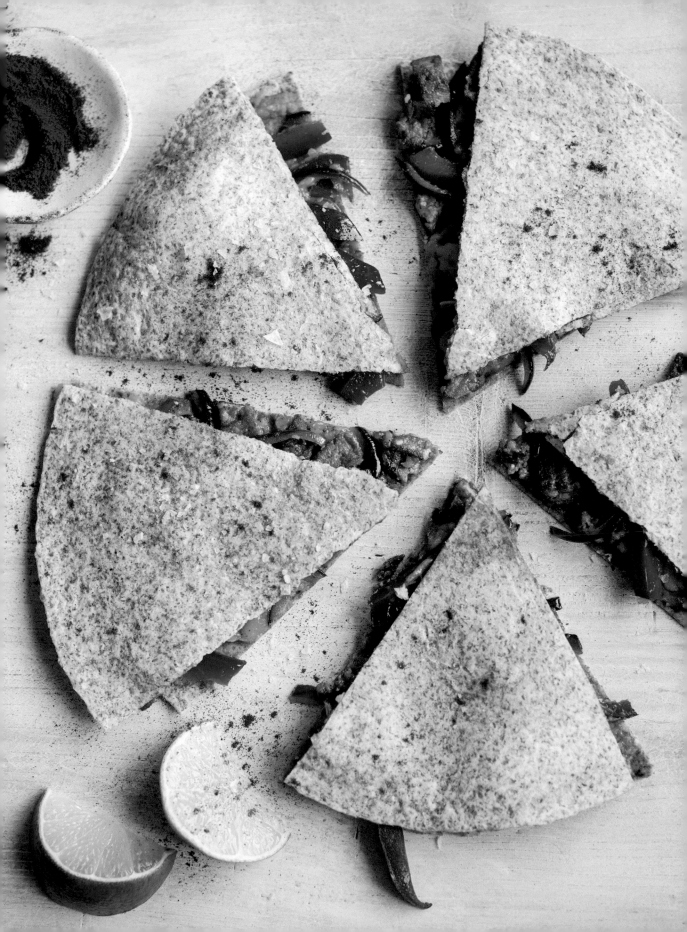

MUSCLE-BUILDING

CALORIES: 632
Protein: 39g
Fat: 15g
Carb: 86g

Jacket Potato with Protein Cheese and Beans

SERVES 1

This is a great way for vegetarians to get a high-carb, high-protein meal in.

1 large jacket potato
200g baked beans
(homemade see page 182
or ½ × 400g tin)
1 tbsp butter
2 large handfuls grated Eat
Lean Protein Cheese

A jacket potato is a great, easy meal for a muscle-building goal. Cheese and beans is a classic combo but you could also try Greek Cottage Cheese (see page 150) or Tuna Salad (see page 146).

1. Preheat the oven to 200°C/Fan 180°C.

2. Prick the potato deeply and evenly with a fork, or score it in a cross pattern. Place in the oven and cook for 45–60 minutes, until soft. (Alternatively, you can cook in a microwave on high for about 9 minutes.)

3. Just before the potato is ready, heat the beans in a saucepan over a medium heat for 5–6 minutes.

4. Remove the potato from the oven, open it up with a knife, then mash in the butter with a fork. Season well with salt and freshly ground black pepper.

5. Top the potato with half the grated cheese, then pour over the beans. Finish with the remaining cheese and serve.

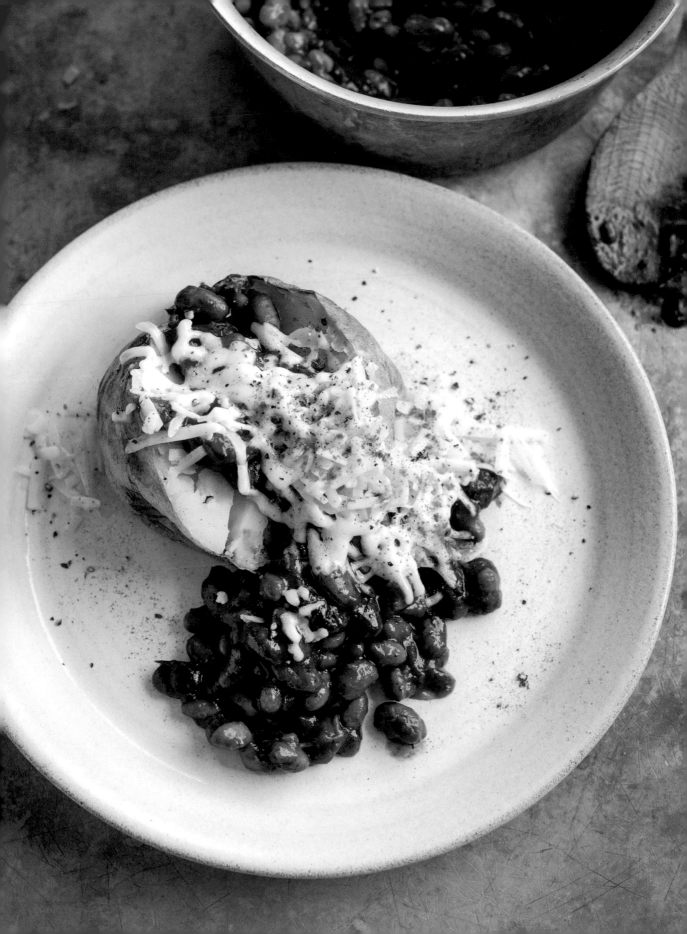

MUSCLE-BUILDING

CALORIES: 573
Protein: 39g
Fats: 30g
Carbs: 38g

Vegan Sunday Roast

SERVES 1

Here's a vegan twist on the British staple!

1 baking potato, peeled
  and quartered
1 small packet firm tofu
  (approx. 200g)
1 tbsp olive oil
1 tsp paprika
1 large handful frozen peas,
  or any greens you prefer
  (spinach, kale or broccoli)
1 tbsp vegetable gravy
  granules

1. Preheat the oven to 200°C/Fan 180°C.

2. Bring a small saucepan of salted water to the boil
and add the potato. Cook for 20 minutes, then drain
and place on kitchen paper to cool for a few minutes.

3. Meanwhile, press the tofu by wrapping it in paper
towels and placing it under a heavy object (like a
chopping board) for 20 minutes. This will reduce
some of the moisture.

4. Cut the pressed tofu into 2 thick slices and place
on a baking tray. Arrange the potato quarters
alongside and, using the kitchen towel, gently
squish them down with your hand.

5. Drizzle the olive oil over the tofu and spuds, and
season well with salt, freshly ground black pepper
and paprika. Roast in the oven for 20 minutes.

6. Remove the tray from the oven, turn the tofu
and spuds, season again, then cook for a further
20 minutes.

7. Meanwhile, bring a small pan of salted water to
the boil and cook the peas and kale for 4–5 minutes
over a medium heat. Drain the veg and pour the
cooking water into a small jug, add the gravy
granules and stir to make the gravy.

8. Plate up and serve.

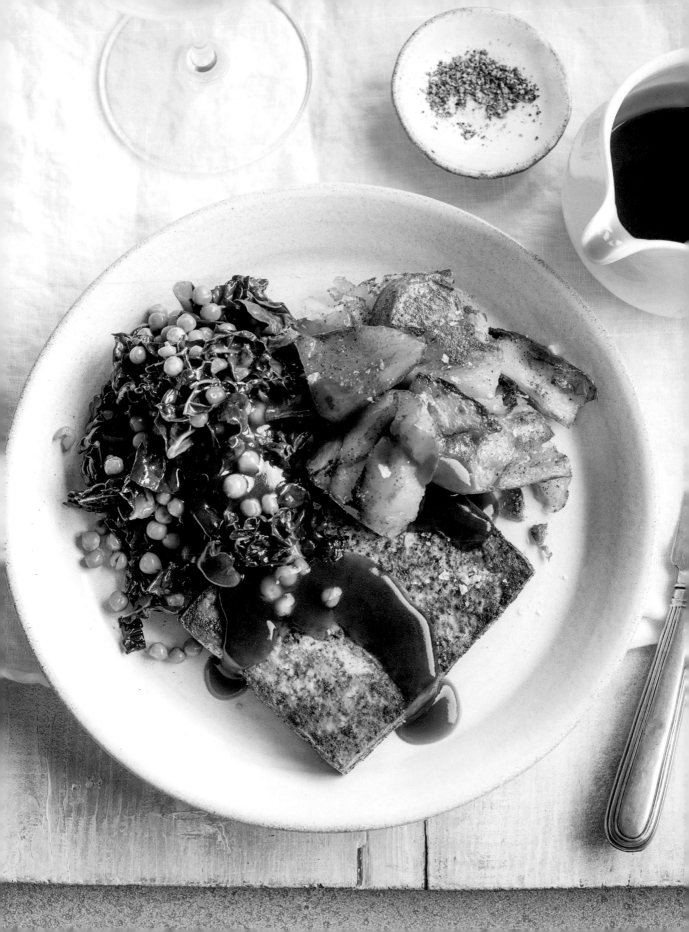

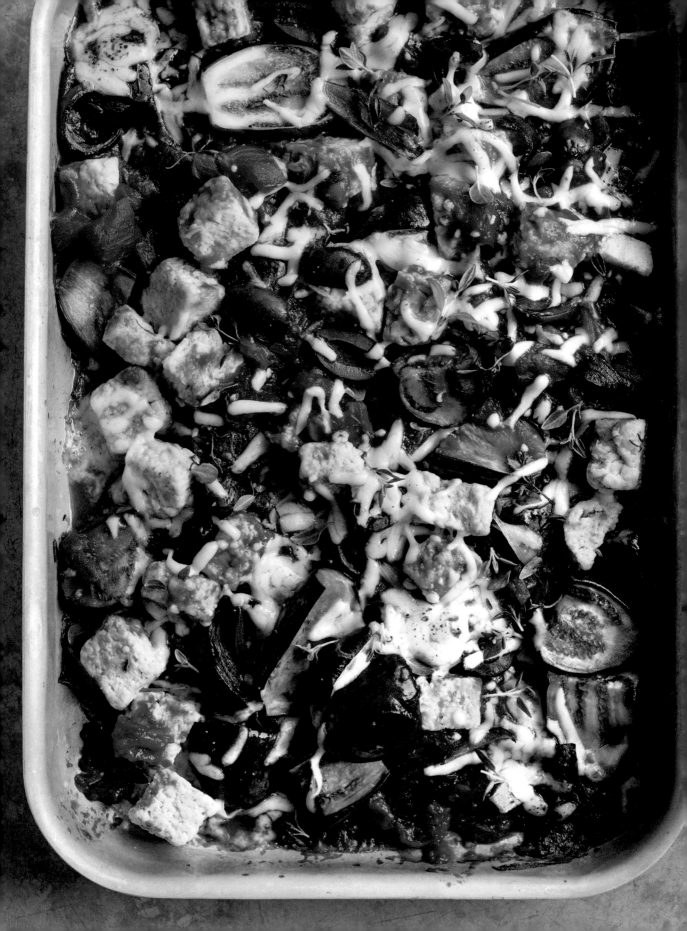

CALORIES: 594
Protein: 42.5g
Fats: 27.4g
Carbs: 35.2g

Protein Traybake

SERVES 1

This traybake is vegetarian but you could swap the Quorn for pieces of chicken breast, pork fillet or fish. You could even leave the protein out of the traybake and serve the roasted veg with a steak instead. The combination of roasted aubergine, tomato, olives and mozzarella goes well with pretty much anything.

½ onion (any), peeled and sliced
1 garlic clove, peeled and crushed
1 large aubergine, cut into large chunks, or 2 small aubergines, halved
1 tbsp olive oil
1 × 400g tin chopped tomatoes
200g Quorn pieces
handful black olives, halved
½ tsp dried oregano or thyme (or 2 tsp fresh)
1 handful grated mozzarella

1. Preheat the oven to 200°C/Fan 180°C.

2. Place the onion, garlic and aubergine on a baking tray. Drizzle over the olive oil and season with salt and freshly ground black pepper. Cook in the oven for 8–10 minutes, until the aubergine has started to colour.

3. Remove the tray from the oven and turn the aubergine. Stir in the tomatoes, Quorn, olives and oregano or thyme. Scatter over the mozzarella and return to the oven for 10–15 minutes.

4. Check the seasoning and serve.

This recipe is easily adapted for vegans by using vegan cheese instead of mozzarella.

MUSCLE-BUILDING

CALORIES: 696
Protein: 37g
Fats: 33g
Carbs: 60g

 # Chilli Prawn Pasta

SERVES 1

This dish works well with pretty much any seafood, so feel free to switch it up!

1 large handful fresh
   spaghetti (or 60g dried)
2 tbsp olive oil
1 tsp chopped, crushed
   or puréed garlic
½ tsp chopped fresh chilli
1 small packet raw prawns
   (approx. 150g)
3 tbsp roughly chopped
   fresh parsley

1. Bring a saucepan of salted water to the boil and cook the spaghetti according to the packet instructions.

2. Meanwhile, heat 1 tablespoon of the olive oil in a frying pan over a high heat. Add the garlic and chilli and, as soon as the oil starts to spit, stir in the prawns so they pick up the other flavours.

3. Drain the spaghetti and return to the saucepan.

4. As soon as the prawns are pink, pour the entire contents of the frying pan over the spaghetti, add the parsley and stir everything together well.

5. Add the remaining olive oil, season well with salt and freshly ground black pepper and serve.

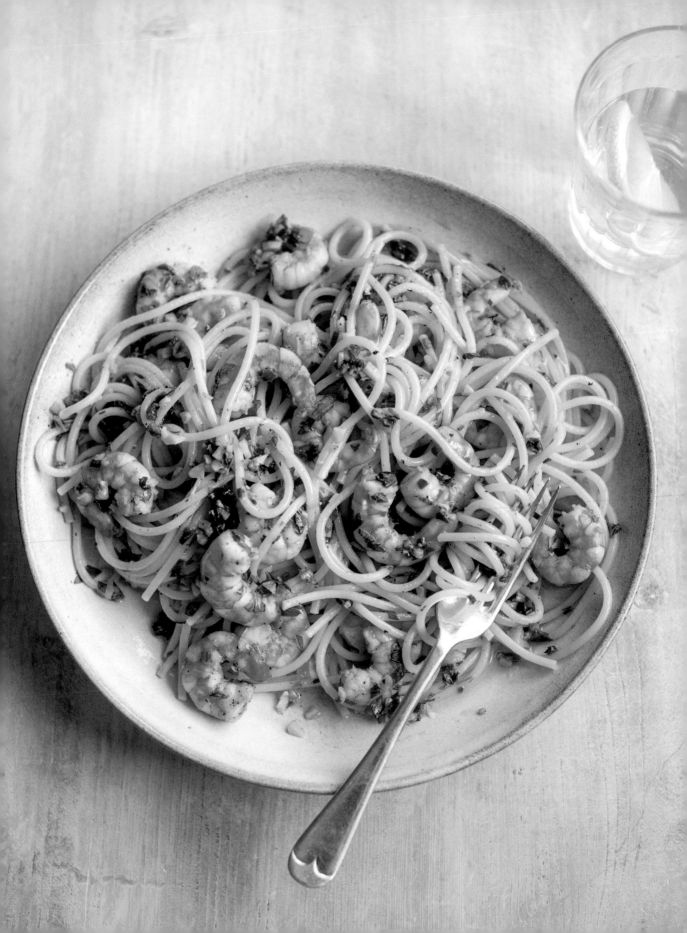

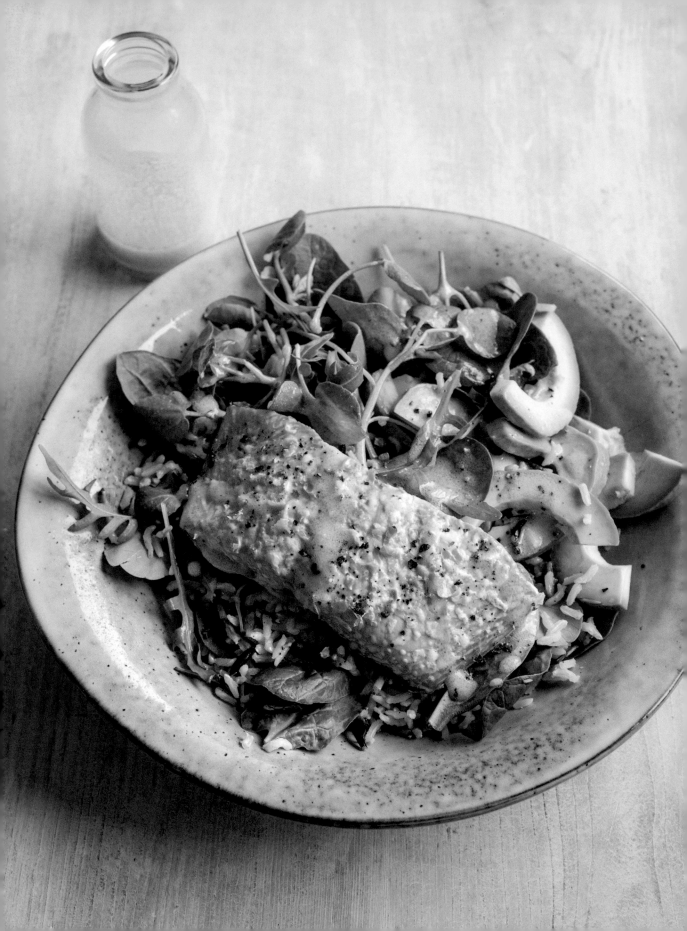

Grilled Salmon Wholegrain Salad

SERVES 1

Salmon is a great double whammy of protein and fat, and when coupled with a big bowl of wholegrains and leaves, you simply cannot get a healthier plate of food.

1 fillet salmon
   (typically 120g)
1 lemon
1 bowl salad leaves (I like
   rocket and spinach here;
   the peppery leaves are
   fantastic with salmon)
½ small avocado, sliced
1 tsp Dijon mustard
1 tbsp olive oil
1 packet microwavable
   brown or wild rice rice
   (approx. 250g)

1. Preheat the grill to high.

2. Place the salmon on a baking tray and squeeze half the lemon juice and grate some zest over the top (it doesn't need any oil or butter as the fish is oily enough already). Season well with salt and freshly ground black pepper.

3. Grill the salmon for 10–15 minutes (the time will depend on the size of the fillet).

4. Meanwhile, place the salad leaves in a bowl and top with the avocado slices.

5. Squeeze the rest of the lemon juice into a cup, add the Dijon mustard and mix well with the olive oil, seasoning with salt and freshly ground black pepper. Drizzle the dressing over the salad.

6. Microwave the rice for 2–3 minutes.

7. Shake the rice out over the salad, then top with the salmon. Drizzle any cooking juices over the top, check the seasoning and serve.

CALORIES: 797
Protein: 40g
Fats: 48g
Carbs: 51g

Salad Niçoise with a Kick

SERVES 1

This is a super-healthy, super-macro-friendly way to get your calories in!

5 new potatoes
2 small eggs
1 tuna steak (approx. 120g)
2 tbsp chilli oil
1 large bowl mixed salad
  leaves (any)
¼ red onion, peeled and
  thinly sliced
1 tbsp balsamic vinegar

COOK'S
TIP

You can make your own chilli oil by placing 450ml olive oil in a saucepan over a gentle heat. Add 1 heaped tablespoon of dried chilli flakes and 3 whole chillies. Warm gently for 3–4 minutes then remove from the heat and leave to cool. Pour into a sterilised bottle and keep for a week in the fridge.

1. Bring a large saucepan of salted water to the boil. Place the potatoes and eggs in the pan and cook over a medium-high heat for 15–20 minutes. (This will hard boil the eggs. If you like them runnier, add them to the pan 5 minutes before the spuds are done.)

2. Meanwhile, place a non-stick frying pan over a high heat. Season the tuna with salt and freshly ground black pepper and drizzle with 1 tablespoon of the chilli oil. Cook in the pan for 2–3 minutes on each side, until it is flakey (not pink).

3. Place the salad leaves in a bowl and add the red onion.

4. Drain the spuds and cut them in half. Shell the eggs and halve them, too. Slice the tuna steak then add everything to the salad.

5. Drizzle over the remaining tablespoon of chilli oil and the balsamic vinegar, check the seasoning and serve.

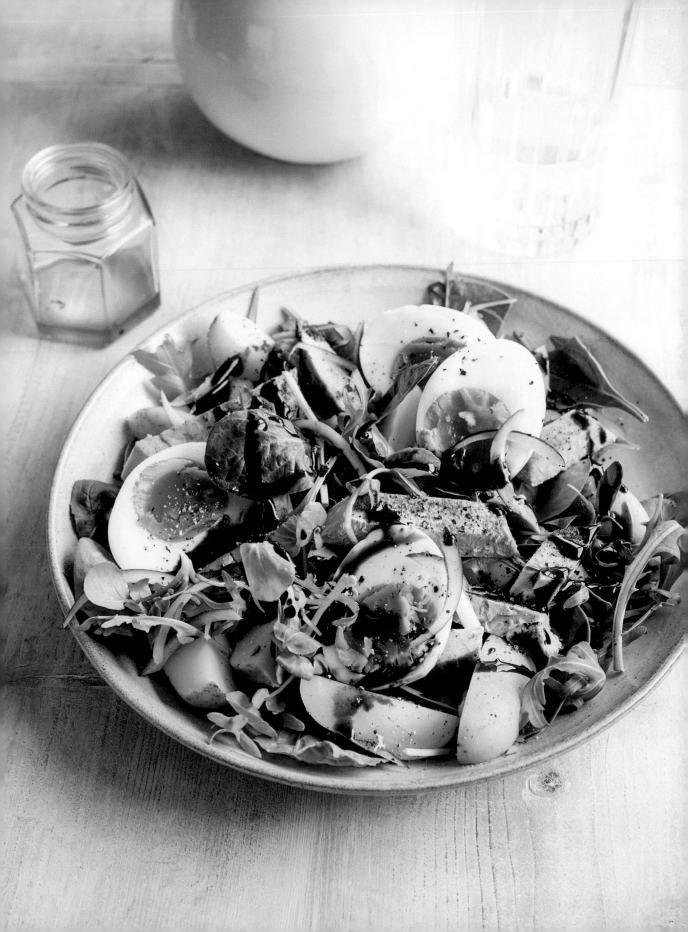

CALORIES: 714
Protein: 43g
Fats: 43g
Carbs: 36g

Quick and Simple Carbonara

SERVES 1

Another meal that feels like an indulgence but meets your calorie, protein, carb and fat goals in one quick cook!

1 small handful lardons
1 large handful fresh
   spaghetti (or 60g dried)
1 large egg
100ml light single cream
2 tbsp grated Parmesan
1 tbsp chopped fresh chives
   (optional)

COOK'S TIP

Make sure to mix the sauce in, plate up and eat this fairly quickly, as the egg will cook over the hot pasta and if you leave it too long it will scramble!

1. Place a non-stick frying pan over a high heat, add the lardons and fry for 5–10 minutes until crispy.

2. Meanwhile, bring a saucepan of salted water to the boil and cook the spaghetti according to the packet instructions.

3. Whisk the egg, cream and 1 tablespoon of the Parmesan together in a bowl.

4. Drain the spaghetti and reserve a small amount of the cooking water. Return both to the pan.

5. Tip the lardons into the pan with the spaghetti, immediately followed by the egg, cream and cheese mixture. Season with salt and freshly ground black pepper and mix together well with a fork.

6. Plate up, top with the remaining Parmesan and sprinkle with chives, if using, to serve.

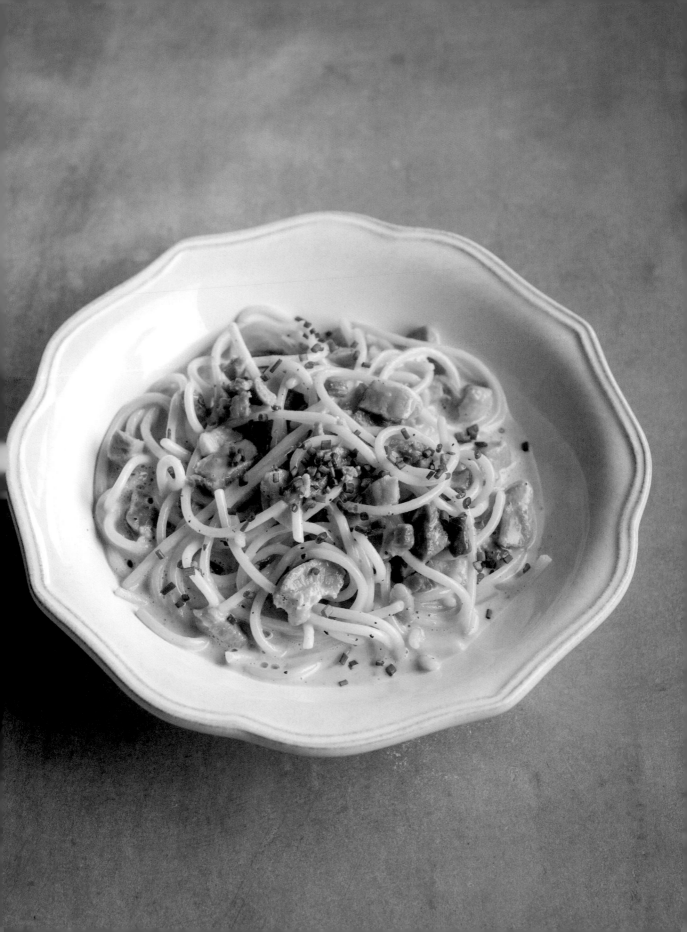

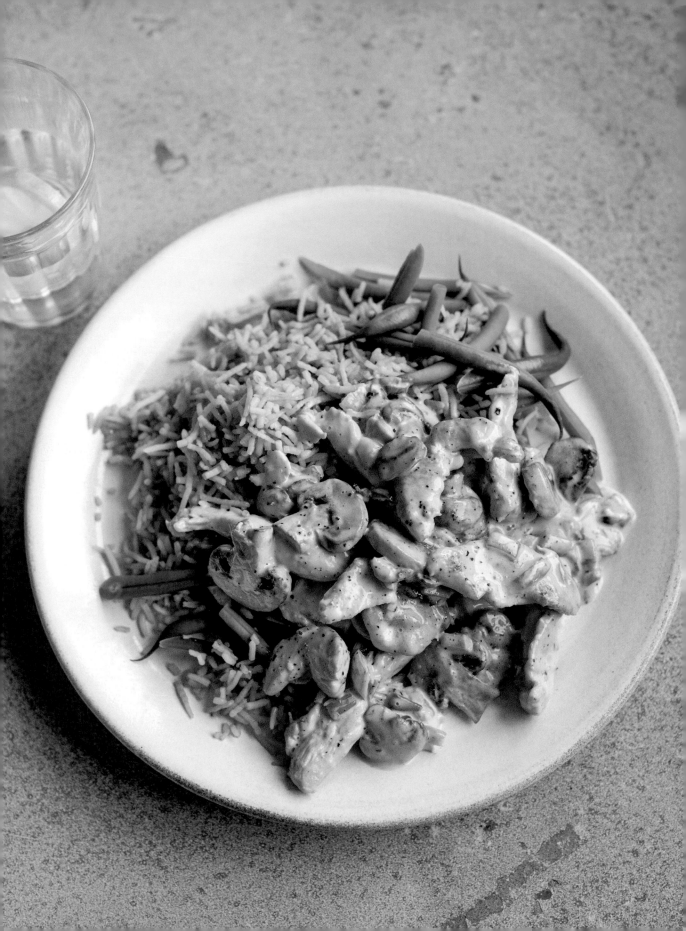

Creamy Chicken and Mushroom Rice

SERVES 1

This feels indulgent but if you have a muscle-building or performance goal, it's a macro-friendly way to get those calories in. This is great served with some steamed green beans or spinach.

1 chicken breast (typically 125–150g), sliced
1 level tbsp salted butter
½ small white onion, peeled and finely chopped
1 tsp chopped, crushed or puréed garlic
1 large handful mushrooms, halved or sliced
100ml light single cream (any)
1 packet microwave wholegrain rice (approx. 250g)

1. Place a non-stick frying pan over a medium heat, add the chicken breast and fry for 6–8 minutes, stirring often, until cooked through. Remove from the pan and set aside.

2. Add the butter to the pan and, when it has melted, add the onion and cook for 2–3 minutes. Add the garlic and mushrooms and continue to cook for 4–5 minutes, until brown.

3. Season the mushrooms and onion well with salt and freshly ground black pepper then reduce the heat to low. Return the chicken to the pan, pour in the cream and stir well.

4. Allow the creamy mushroom sauce to simmer very gently for about 4–5 minutes.

5. Meanwhile, cook the rice in the microwave according to the packet instructions. Tip into a bowl and season well.

6. Top the rice with the chicken and mushrooms then pour over the creamy sauce. Check the seasoning and serve.

MUSCLE-BUILDING

CALORIES: 635
Protein: 50g
Fats: 42g
Carbs: 29g

My Steak Baguette

SERVES 1

Once upon a time this was my favourite lunch, so I have rejigged it for gains!

1 level tbsp butter
1 small fillet steak
(typically 200g)
2 level tbsp mayonnaise
1 tsp mustard
1 small baguette (approx.
15cm long)
1 small handful rocket
¼ red onion, peeled and
thinly sliced

1. Place a non-stick frying pan over a high heat, add the butter and, when it has melted, add the steak to the pan, quickly searing on one side then the other.

2. Reduce the heat a little, season the steak with salt and freshly ground black pepper and cook for 4 minutes on each side (for a medium-rare steak). Remove from the pan and leave to rest.

3. Meanwhile, mix the mayo and mustard together in a small bowl.

4. Slice the baguette lengthways, spread the mayonnaise mix on both sides, then add the rocket and onion to one half.

5. Cut the steak into thin slices and place them on top of the rocket and onion. Cover with the other half of the baguette and serve.

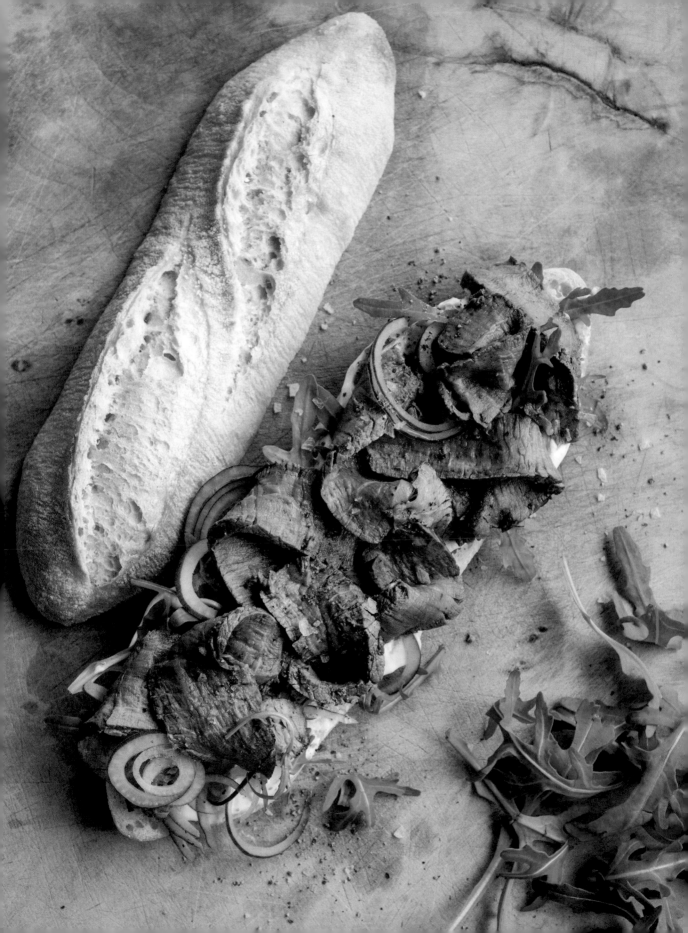

GENERAL HEALTH AND FITNESS GOALS
(well-balanced calorie and macro recipes)

General health and fitness goals should have a happy dietary balance of calories and macronutrients, which is exactly what I have tried to cater to in these recipes.

Please note: Regardless of goals, I ALWAYS recommend carbohydrate consumption pre- and post-workout. If your lunch or dinner is pre- or post-workout, I advise you choose a higher carb recipe both before and after your session.

Vegan Pitta

SERVES 1

This is a very healthy, high-carb, high-fat, high-protein meal!

¼ packet Quorn Vegan
   Fajita Strips (approx. 70g)
1 wholegrain pitta
4 heaped tbsp hummus
½ tomato, finely sliced
1 large handful lettuce (and
   any green leaves you like
   – I love rocket in this),
   roughly chopped
1 tbsp chilli oil (see page
   110 on how to make
   your own)

1. Place a non-stick frying pan over a medium heat and cook the Quorn strips for 5–6 minutes.

2. Meanwhile, toast the pitta, cut in half and spread 2 tablespoons of hummus on each side. Lay the tomato and lettuce slices evenly over the top.

3. Spoon the Quorn strips into the pitta halves and drizzle with the chilli oil.

4. Season with salt and freshly ground black pepper and serve.

CALORIES: 542
Protein: 23g
Fats: 19g
Carbs: 69g

Black Bean Burrito

SERVES 1

This isn't JUST for vegans – the combination of black beans and wholegrains form a complete protein, as well as a great hit of fibre, which is pivotal to gut health!

½ small red pepper, diced
½ small onion (any), peeled and diced
½ × 400g tin black beans, drained and rinsed
1 tsp chopped, crushed or puréed garlic
1 tsp paprika
1 slice vegan cheese or 15g grated
1 wholewheat or seeded tortilla
½ small avocado, thinly sliced
½ tomato, finely sliced
1 tbsp salsa (homemade see page 180 or shop-bought)

1. Place a non-stick frying pan over a medium heat.

2. Add the pepper and onion and cook for a few minutes. Add the black beans, along with the garlic and paprika. Season with salt and freshly ground black pepper.

3. Allow the veg and beans to soften in the pan for 4–5 minutes, stirring frequently.

4. Place the cheese on the tortilla and warm in the microwave on high for about 30 seconds.

5. Remove from the microwave and top with the beans and veg. Place the avocado, tomato and salsa inside the wrap. Fold the bottom end over the filling, then tightly roll using your fingers, from one side to the other.

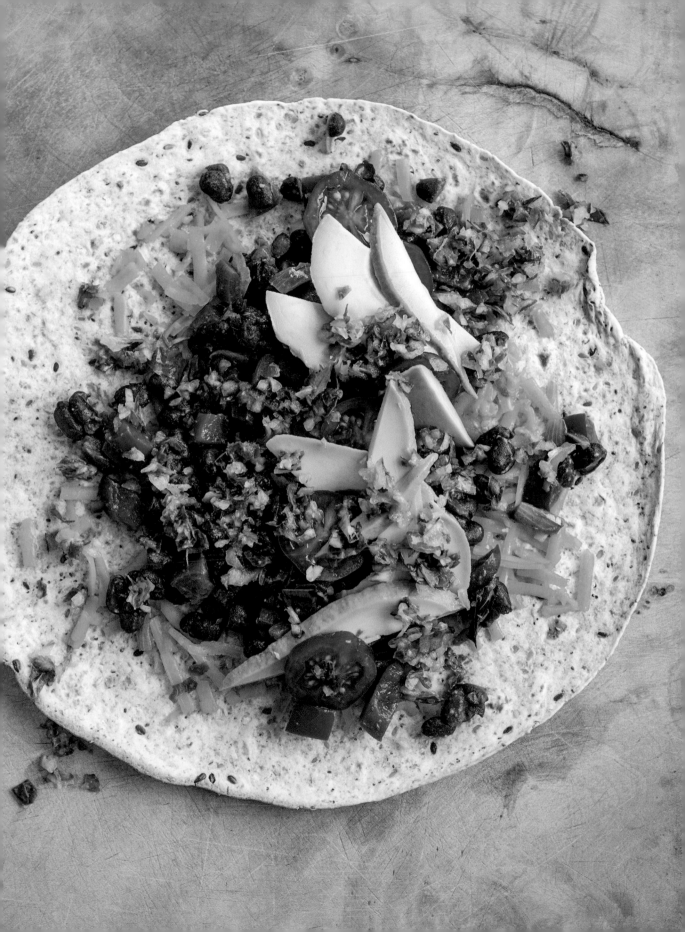

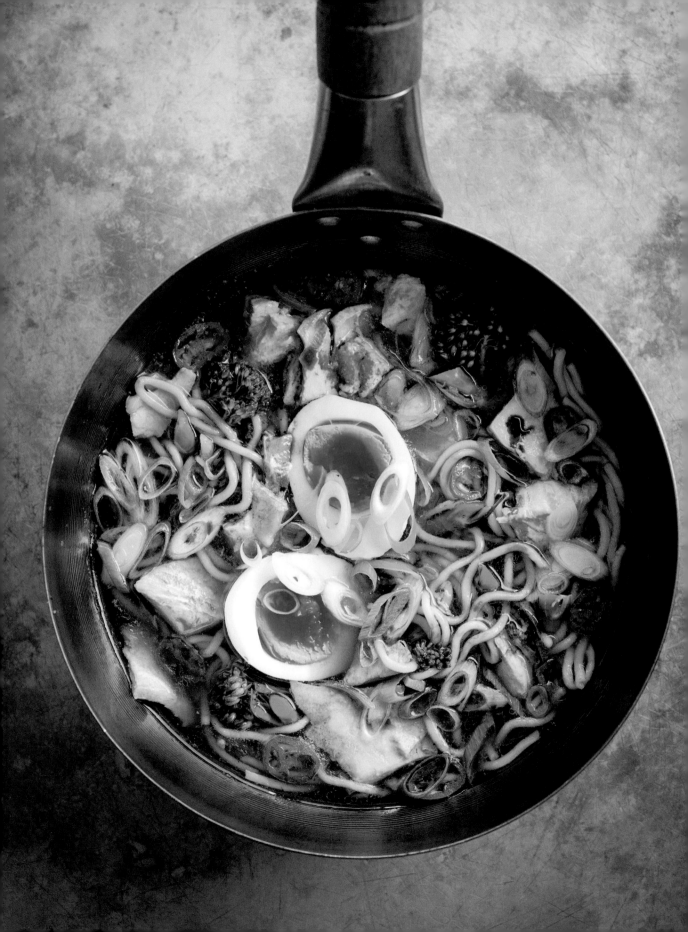

Salmon Ramen

SERVES 1

Pork is the traditional meat in ramen, but for a health-minded cook, oily fish is always a preferable fat and protein combo.

1 tsp sesame oil
1 tbsp chopped, crushed
    or puréed garlic
1 fresh chilli, sliced
1 salmon fillet (typically
    120g), sliced
1 spring onion, finely sliced
1 large handful fresh
    noodles
1 small egg
2 tbsp light soy sauce
2 handfuls green veg
    (I like adding spinach
    and broccoli)

This recipe is easily adapted for vegetarians by using two eggs or 80g tofu instead of the salmon.

COOK'S
TIP

The egg will be very soft-boiled so if you prefer it to be hard, boil it in the pan for a few minutes before adding the noodles.

1. Put the kettle on to boil.

2. Meanwhile, place the sesame oil in a wok or large non-stick frying pan over a high heat and add the garlic and chilli. When the oil starts to spit, add the salmon and fry for 4–5 minutes, tossing frequently, until the fish starts to pink.

3. Pour approximately 500–600ml boiling water from the kettle into the wok (the pan should be about ⅓ full). Immediately add the spring onion, noodles, whole egg (in its shell) and a tablespoon of the soy sauce, as well as any green veg you may want to use.

4. The noodles should take about 4–5 minutes to cook, at which point remove the egg using a spoon, and pour the ramen into a large bowl.

5. Hold the egg under the cold tap and gently remove and discard the shell. Halve the egg and place on top of the ramen bowl. Season with another tablespoon of soy sauce and serve.

CALORIES: 411
Protein: 44g
Fats: 11g
Carbs: 33g

Ratatouille Cod

SERVES 1

I used to make this as a teenager when I briefly tried (and failed) the Atkins diet. However, this is SUCH a healthy recipe that it has long since stayed a favourite!

½ onion (any), peeled and sliced
½ large courgette, sliced
½ red pepper, sliced
1 large handful mushrooms, sliced
½ × 400g tin chopped tomatoes
1 tsp chopped, crushed or puréed garlic
2–3 fresh basil leaves, shredded
1 fillet cod (typically 120g)
½ lemon
2 level tbsp grated Parmesan

1. Preheat the oven to 200°C/Fan 180°C.

2. Place the onion, courgette, pepper and mushrooms in an oven dish. Pour over the tinned tomatoes and stir in the garlic and basil. Season with salt and freshly ground black pepper and bake in the oven for 10 minutes.

3. Remove the tray from the oven and turn the veg. Place the cod fillet on top, squeeze over the lemon and season the fish well. Bake in the oven for 15 minutes.

4. Remove from the oven, sprinkle over the Parmesan and serve.

This recipe is easily adapted for vegetarians by using Quorn or tofu instead of cod.

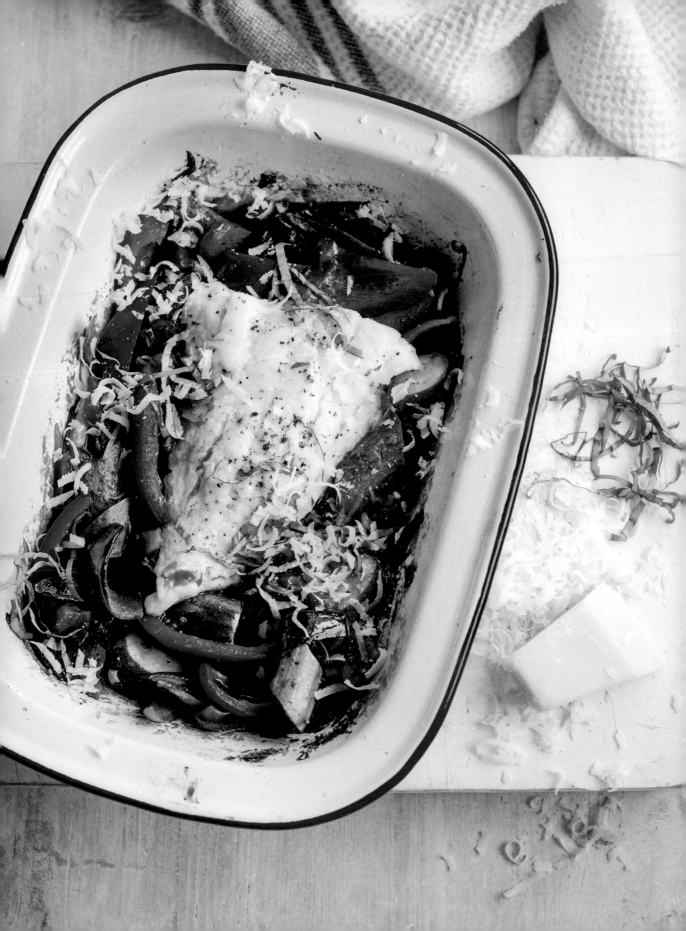

GENERAL HEALTH

CALORIES: 523
Protein: 44g
Fats: 25g
Carbs: 30g

Tuna Pasta with an Upgrade!

SERVES 1

This is a great way to get a hit of protein, fats, carbs and fibre.

1 large handful fresh penne
  or fusilli pasta
1 tuna steak (approx. 120g)
1 level tbsp full-fat
  mayonnaise
1 large handful tinned
  sweetcorn
1 large handful spinach
1 small handful grated
  Cheddar
1 tbsp chopped fresh chives
  (optional)

1. Bring a saucepan of salted water to the boil and cook the pasta according to the packet instructions.

2. Meanwhile, place a non-stick frying pan over a high heat. Season the tuna with salt and freshly ground black pepper then cook in the pan for 2–3 minutes on each side, until it is flakey (not pink).

3. Drain the pasta and reserve a little of the cooking water. Return both to the pan.

4. Add the tuna, mayonnaise and sweetcorn to the pan. Stir everything together well so the tuna breaks up and the mayo coats the pasta. Check the seasoning.

5. Place the spinach in the bottom of a large bowl, top with the tuna pasta, sprinkle over the cheese and chives, if using, and serve.

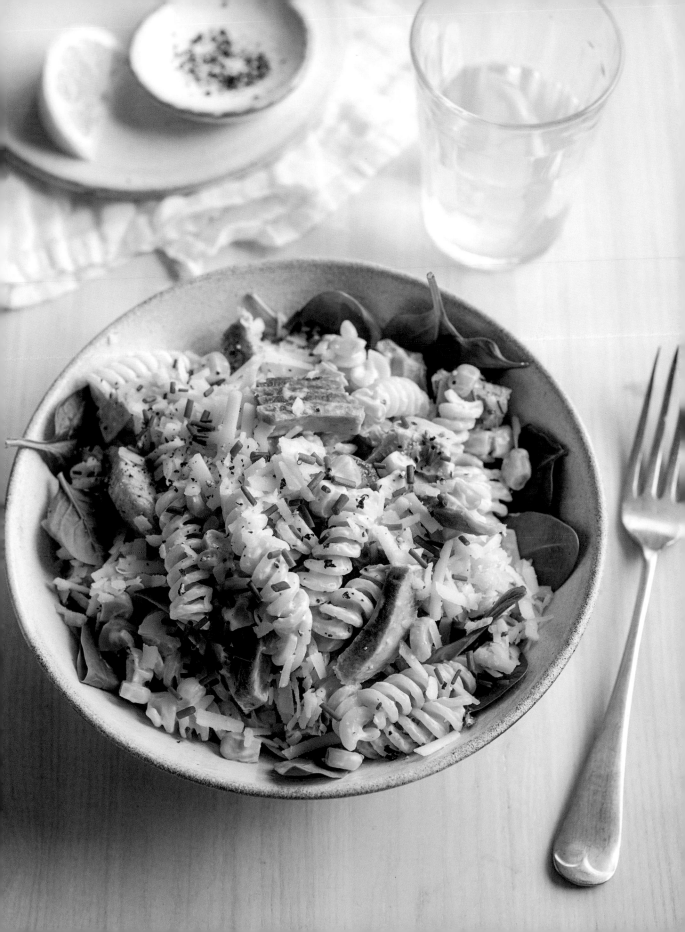

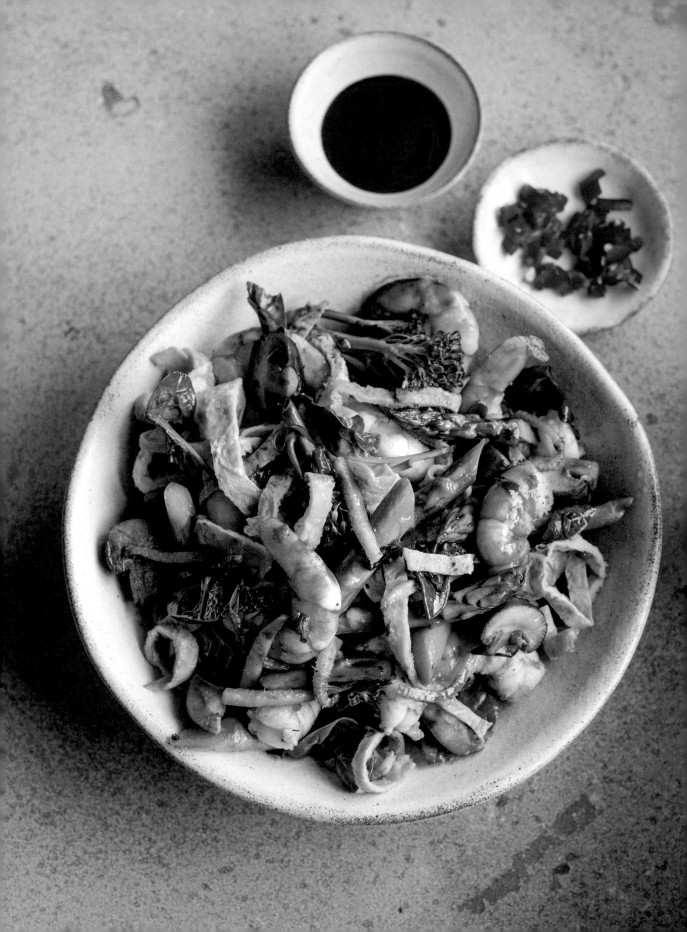

Prawn Stir Fry

SERVES 1

Proteins, fats, carbs, micronutrients and fibre – what more do you need?

1 tbsp sesame oil
1 tbsp chopped, crushed
   or puréed garlic
1 chilli, finely chopped
1 tbsp thinly sliced (or
   chopped) fresh ginger
1 small packet raw prawns
   (approx. 150g)
1 large handful
   mushrooms, halved
   or quartered
1 large handful broccoli
   florets
1 large handful asparagus
   spears, cut into lengths
1 large handful spinach
   leaves
2 tbsp light soy sauce
2 small eggs, beaten

This recipe is easily
adapted for vegetarians
by using Quorn or tofu
instead of prawns.

1. Place the sesame oil in a wok or large non-stick frying pan over a high heat. Add the garlic, chilli and ginger and, when the oil starts to spit, chuck in the prawns and cook for 1–2 minutes, tossing so they turn pink evenly.

2. Add all the veg and toss everything together well. Cook for 3–4 minutes, until the veg have started to soften. Season with a generous tablespoon of soy sauce and toss again.

3. Meanwhile, place the eggs in a separate pan over a medium heat and swirl to cook a thin omelette. Remove from the pan, roll into a tube and cut into thin slices.

4. Plate up the prawns and veg, top with the omelette strips, drizzle with the remaining soy sauce and serve.

GENERAL HEALTH

CALORIES: 444

Protein: 57g
Fats: 17g
Carbs: 16g

Spicy Chicken Salad

SERVES 1

This is a very low-carb, high-protein salad filled to the brim with good fats and micronutrients!

½ small pot 0% Greek yoghurt (approx. 100g)
1 level tbsp peanut butter (homemade see page 183 or shop-bought)
1 tsp curry powder
1 chicken breast (typically 125–150g)
1 large bowl lettuce (any green leaves you like)
½ small red onion, peeled and finely sliced
½ small cucumber, diced
1 large carrot, peeled then grated or peeled into ribbons
1 small handful peanuts (approx. 20g)

This recipe is easily adapted for vegetarians by using Quorn or tofu instead of chicken.

1. Preheat the oven to 220°C/Fan 200°C.

2. Mix the yoghurt, peanut butter and curry powder in a small bowl. Place half the mixture in a separate larger bowl and add the chicken breast, covering it generously in the sauce.

3. Make a bed out of tinfoil and place the chicken breast in the centre, spooning any remaining marinade over the chicken. Cook in the oven for 20–30 minutes, until the juices run clear.

4. Meanwhile, to make the salad, place the lettuce in a large bowl and add the onion, cucumber and carrot, mixing well.

5. Slice the chicken and place on top of the salad. Use the reserved yoghurt mixture as a dressing (thinned with a little water, if needed). Sprinkle over the peanuts, season with salt and freshly ground black pepper and serve.

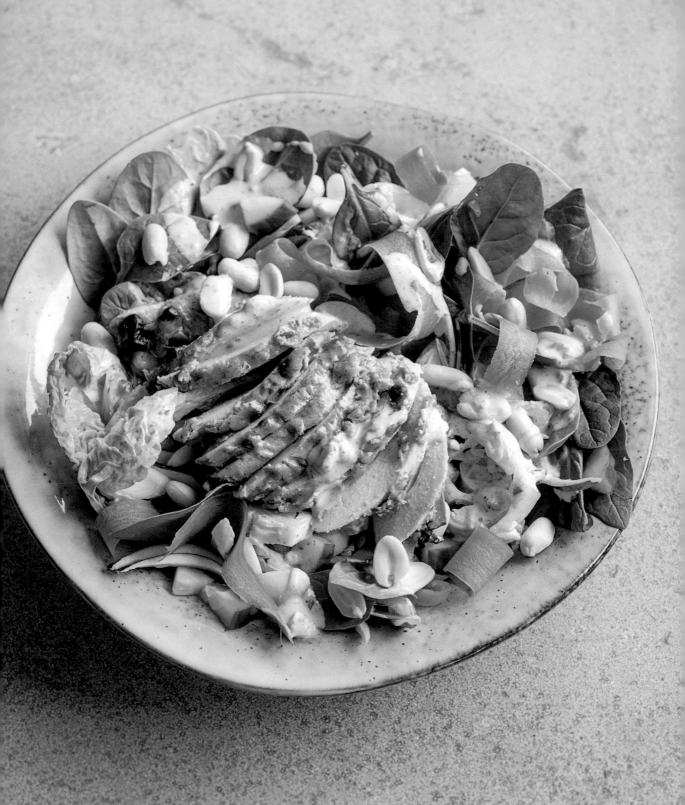

CALORIES: 499
Protein: 52g
Fats: 22g
Carbs: 24g

Herby Lemon Chicken Salad

SERVES 1

A high-protein, high-fat, high-fibre, highly nutritious meal!

1 small pot 0% Greek (or soy) yoghurt (approx. 170g)
½ tsp dried mixed herbs, plus a pinch
zest and juice of 1 lemon
1 chicken breast (typically 125–150g)
½ courgette, roughly chopped
½ pepper, roughly chopped
½ red onion, peeled and roughly chopped
1 large bowl mixed salad leaves (any)
1 tbsp olive oil
1 large handful olives (any)

This recipe is easily adapted for vegetarians by using Quorn or tofu instead of chicken.

1. Heat the oven to 200°C/Fan 180°C.

2. Mix the yoghurt, herbs, lemon zest and half the lemon juice in a small bowl. Place half in a separate larger bowl and add the chicken, coating it well.

3. Make a bed out of tinfoil and place the chicken breast inside it, spooning any remaining marinade over the top. Arrange the pepper, onion and courgette in the tinfoil around the chicken, season well with salt and freshly ground black pepper and cook in the oven for 20–30 minutes, until the chicken juices run clear.

4. Meanwhile, place the salad leaves in a bowl. Dress with the olive oil and the remaining lemon juice and add another pinch of the mixed herbs.

5. Remove the chicken and veg from the oven. Slice the chicken and place on top of the salad with the veg. Sprinkle with the olives and spoon the reserved yoghurt mixture over the top. Check the seasoning and serve.

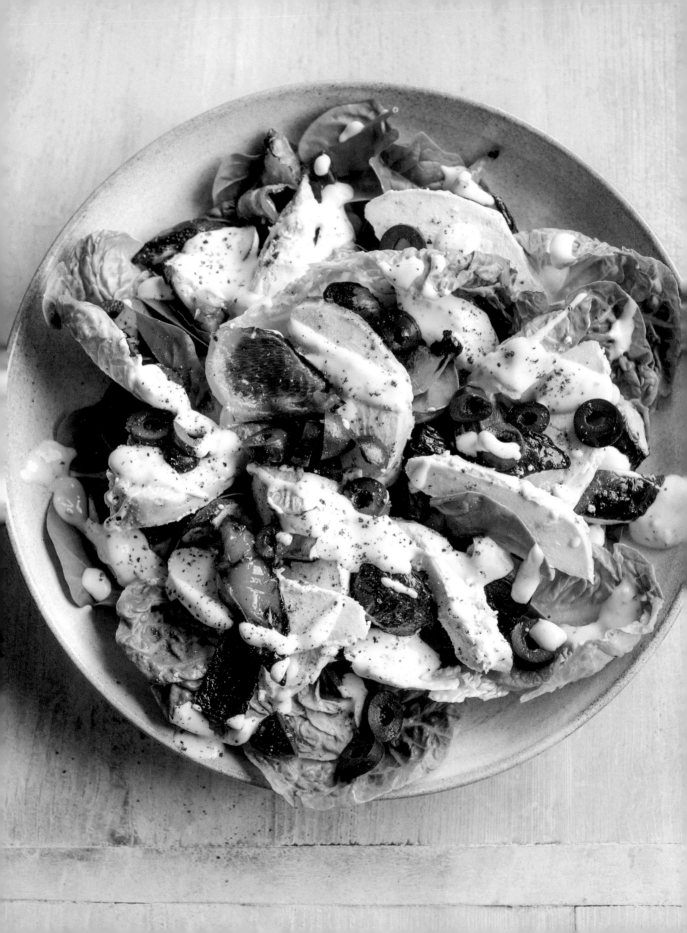

CALORIES: 488
Protein: 28g
Fats: 22g
Carbs: 43g

Spicy Chicken Sausage Pasta

SERVES 1

Spicy sausage pasta is fantastic, but if you have a health goal, sausages probably aren't your best source of fats and proteins. Try lean chicken sausages instead!

1 tbsp olive oil
1 tsp chopped, crushed
    or puréed garlic
1 chilli, sliced
½ white onion, peeled
    and diced
3 Heck chicken chipolatas,
    roughly chopped
½ × 400g tin chopped
    tomatoes
1 large handful fresh
    spaghetti (or 60g dried)
1 handful fresh basil leaves
    (optional)

This recipe is easily adapted for vegetarians by using vegetarian sausages instead of chicken.

1. Place a non-stick frying pan over a high heat and add the oil, garlic and chilli. When the oil starts to spit, add the onion and sausages. Reduce the heat to medium and cook for 5–6 minutes, until the onions have softened and the sausages have browned.

2. Reduce the heat to low and pour in the chopped tomatoes. Season with salt and freshly ground black pepper and stir all the ingredients together well.

3. Meanwhile, bring a saucepan of salted water to the boil and cook the spaghetti according to the packet instructions.

4. Drain the spaghetti and tip it back into the pan. Spoon the contents of the frying pan over the spaghetti and mix together well.

5. Check the seasoning, sprinkle with the basil leaves, if using, and serve.

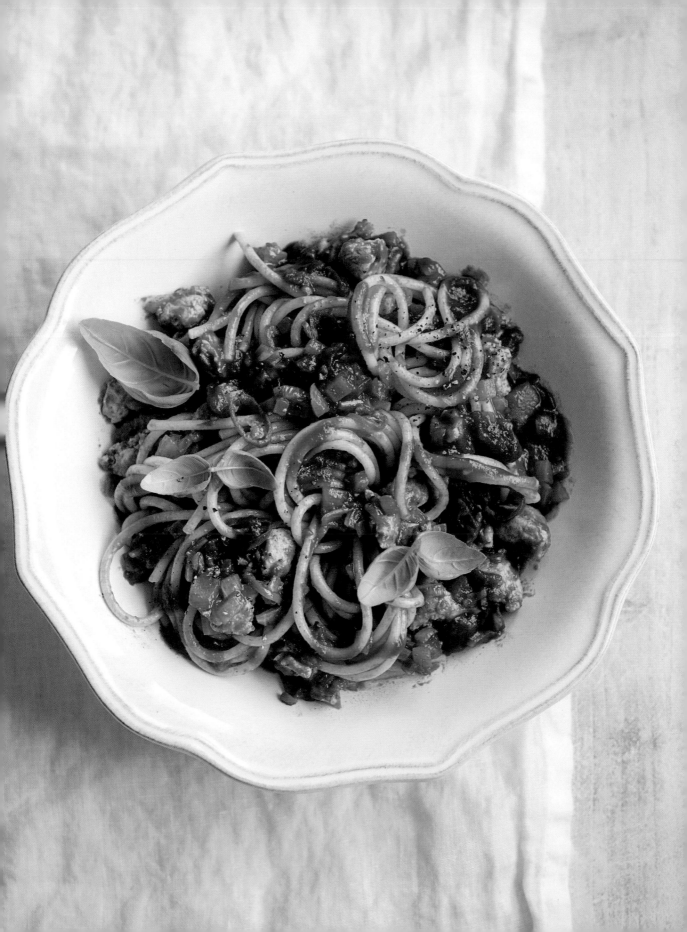

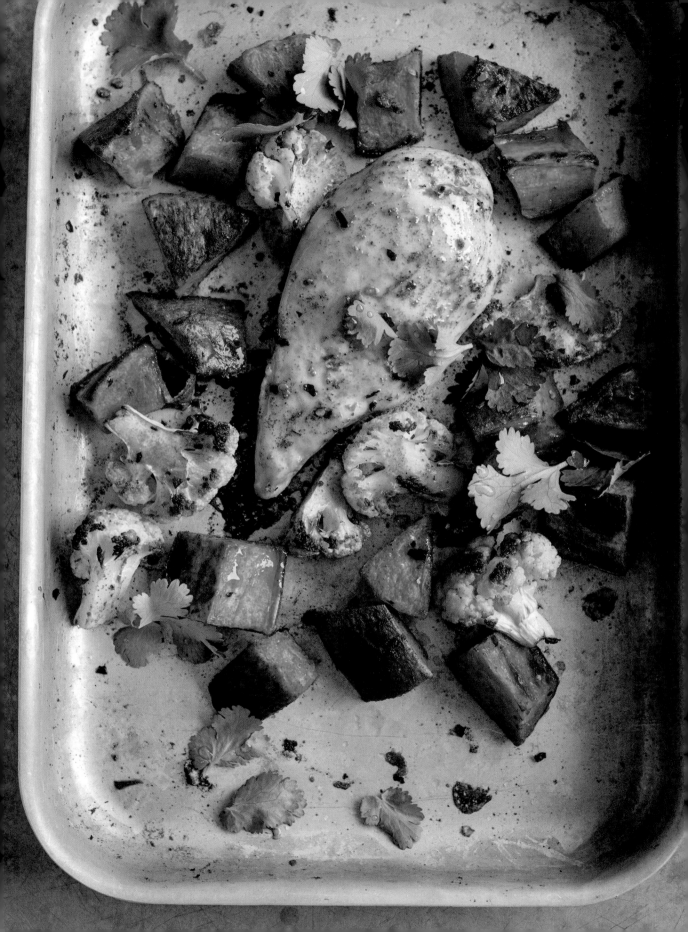

Sweet Potato, Cauliflower, Squash and Chicken Traybake

SERVES 1

A quick and easy meal that is full of protein and healthy carbs.

½ medium sweet potato (typically 100g), peeled and cubed

100g cauliflower, broken into florets

100g butternut squash, peeled and cut into chunks

1 tbsp olive oil

¼ tsp ground cumin

¼ tsp ground turmeric

¼ tsp dried chilli flakes

1 chicken breast (typically 125–150g)

1 handful fresh coriander leaves (optional)

This recipe is easily adapted for vegetarians and vegans by using a Quorn fillet instead of chicken.

1. Preheat the oven to 200°C/Fan 180°C.

2. Place the sweet potato, cauliflower and squash in a large bowl. Drizzle over the olive oil and sprinkle in the spices and chilli. Mix everything together well to coat the veg. Season with salt and freshly ground black pepper.

3. Tip the veg on to a baking tray and cook in the oven for 10 minutes, until they have started to colour.

4. Remove the tray from the oven and turn the veg. Add the chicken and return to the oven for another 20–25 minutes, until the chicken is cooked through.

5. Check the seasoning, sprinkle with coriander, if using, and serve.

GENERAL HEALTH

CALORIES: 569
Protein: 65.8g
Fats: 19.4g
Carbs: 38.6g

Pork Fillet and Cheesy New Potatoes

SERVES 1

Proteins, fats, carbs, fibre and micronutrients – I'm a happy girl when I can tick all five of these boxes!

4 new potatoes
1 tsp paprika
1 small handful grated
  Cheddar
1 small, lean pork fillet
  (typically 175g)
1 large handful kale
1 large handful sliced leeks
1 tsp chopped, crushed
  or puréed garlic

COOK'S TIP

When it comes to healthy cooking, I'd usually recommend fish and chicken over red meat. However, that doesn't mean you always have to go with fish and chicken! There are some great nutrients in beef, pork, lamb and game.

1. Preheat the grill to medium.

2. Bring a saucepan of salted water to the boil and cook the spuds for 15–20 minutes, until tender. Drain and place on a small baking tray.

3. Using the heel of your hand and a kitchen towel, smash the spuds down gently so they break a little and soften. Season well with paprika, salt and freshly ground pepper, then sprinkle over the cheese.

4. Grill for 5–10 minutes, until the cheese has melted and become slightly golden.

5. Meanwhile, place a non-stick frying pan over a high heat. Add the fillet and fry for approximately 6–7 minutes on each side. Remove the pork from the pan and set aside to rest.

6. Using the same frying pan, cook the kale, leeks and garlic over a high heat for 5–6 minutes, until soft.

7. Slice the pork and serve with the spuds and veg.

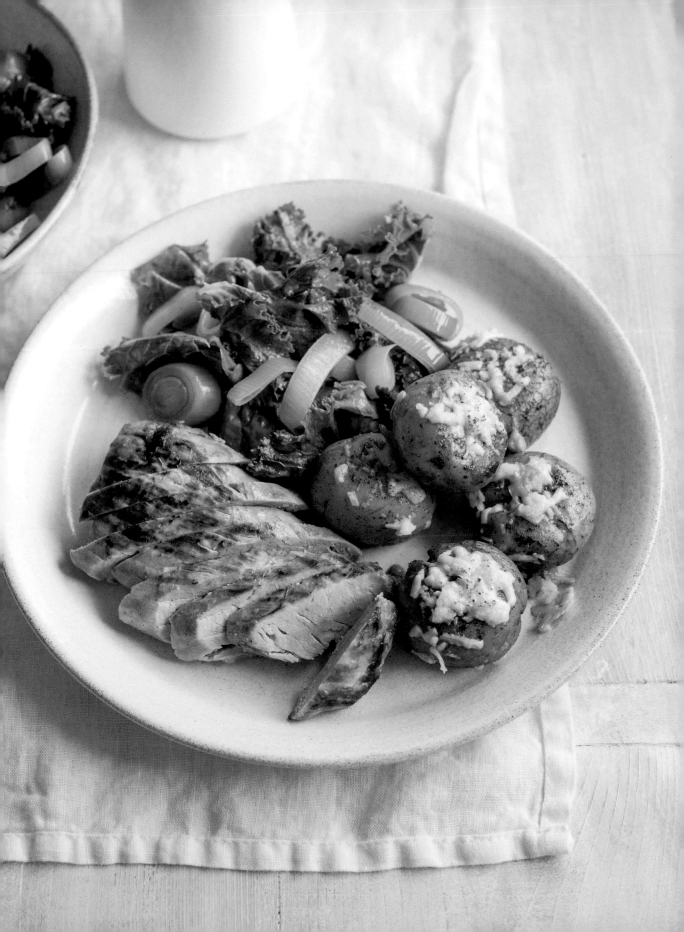

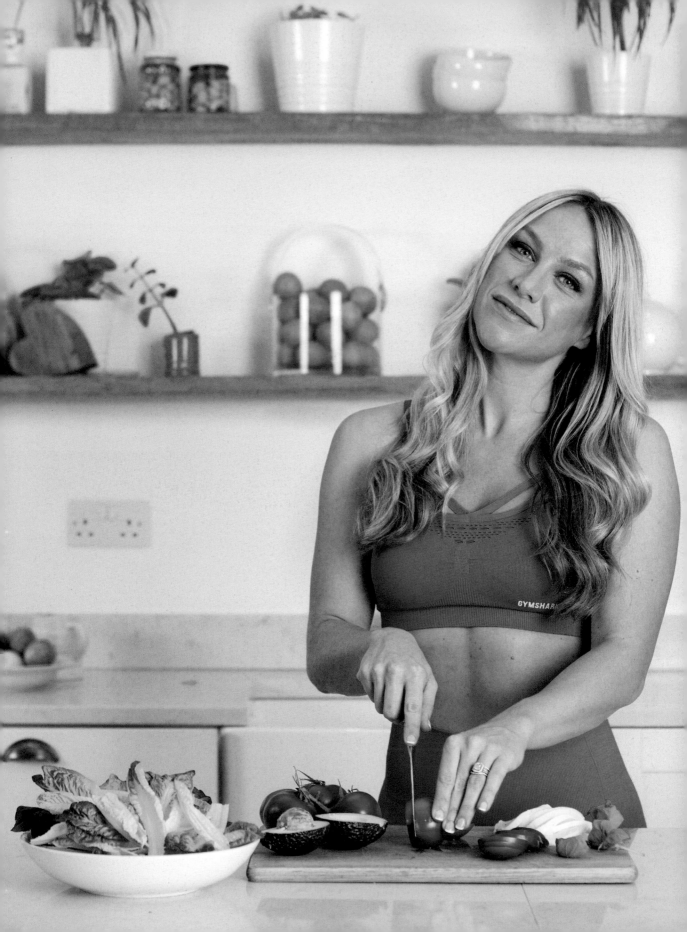

SAVOURY & SWEET SNACKS

○ ● ○

I always get asked for snack recommendations
but, truth be told, I'm not really a big snacker.
That being said, my husband eats more
snacks than he does meals so I had a long,
old catalogue for this section!

SAVOURY & SWEET SNACK RECIPES

In an ideal world, you'd eat calorie- and macro-dense MEALS both pre- and post-training. This ensures your food is going to good use during the training session, and in the anabolic and recovery window thereafter.

These snacks are to help you make up your calories during the rest of the day, and keep both your energy and satiety levels up.

Most of these snacks are high in protein.

All of these snacks are 300kcals and under so are suitable for all goals.

CALORIES: 300
Protein: 10.7g
Fats: 20.1g
Carbs: 18.5g

Cheesy Popcorn

SERVES 1

For those who prefer savoury to sweet!

1 small handful
    popping corn
1 tsp salted butter
1 large handful grated
    Cheddar

COOK'S TIP

A small handful of
popping corn goes
a long way and can
be made much lower
in calories than the
pre-made alternatives.
Definitely a must-buy
for the cupboard!

1. Place the popping corn and butter in a large bowl (the portion will grow significantly when cooked) and season well with salt.

2. Cover the bowl in clingfilm and pierce it several times with a sharp knife.

3. Microwave on high for 2–3 minutes, until the popping has slowed to 5 second intervals.

4. Remove the clingfilm and scatter the grated cheese over the top. Place the bowl back in the microwave for a further 30 seconds until the cheese has melted.

5. Check the seasoning and serve.

CALORIES: 177
Protein: 23g
Fats: 8.1g
Carbs: 4.2g

Egg White Omelette

SERVES 1

A high-protein option for a savoury snacker.

1 tsp salted butter
4 large egg whites (approx.
    120g), whisked until frothy
1 handful grated mozzarella
5 cherry tomatoes, halved
    or quartered
½ jalapeño pepper, sliced
1 tbsp salsa (homemade see
    page 180 or shop-bought)

1. Place the butter in a non-stick frying pan over a medium heat. As it melts, season the whites, then pour them into the pan.

2. Sprinkle with the mozzarella and top with the tomatoes and jalapeño. Continue to cook.

3. When the omelette has little to no liquid left, fold over and plate up.

4. Spoon the salsa on top to serve.

Whisk your egg whites for a good few minutes to make your omelette super fluffy!

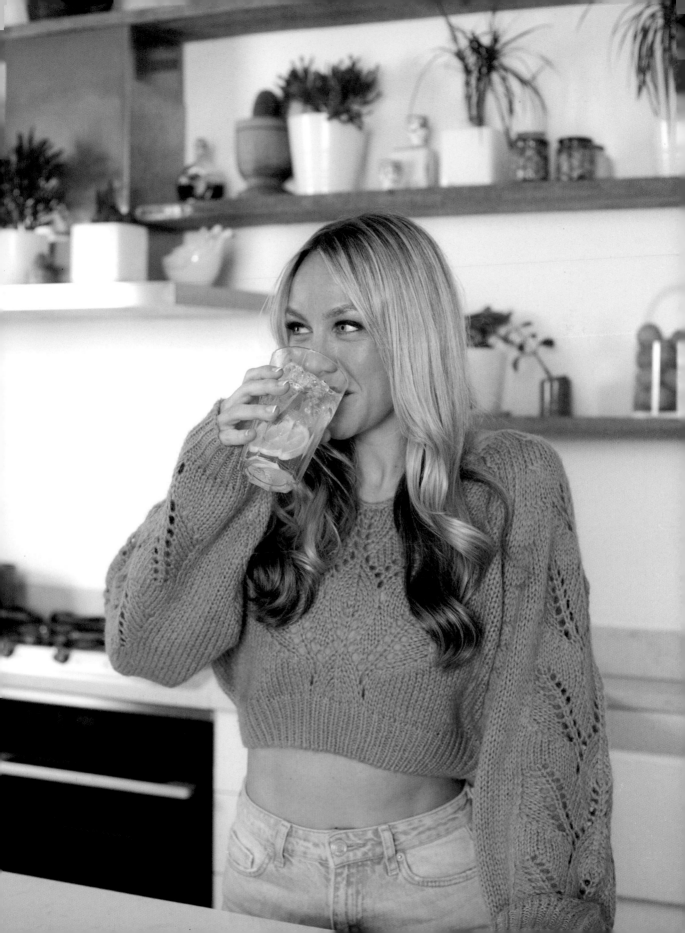

CALORIES: 249
Protein: 20g
Fats: 15.5g
Carbs: 7.5g

Tuna Salad

SERVES 1

A salad can be so low in calories that it can easily be a (very filling) snack!

1 small egg
1 small tin tuna in water
   or brine (approx. 50–60g
   drained weight)
1 level tbsp mayonnaise
1 small handful tinned
   sweetcorn
1 mixed salad bowl (ready-
   made or simply make one
   yourself – just chuck a
   large handful of green
   leaves, such as lettuce
   and spinach, into a bowl
   with some chopped
   tomato, cucumber
   and red onion)

1. Bring a small saucepan of salted water to the boil.

2. Gently lower the egg into the water and cook for 7–8 minutes.

3. Meanwhile, mix the tuna in a bowl with the mayonnaise and sweetcorn.

4. Prepare the mixed salad bowl and spoon the tuna evenly across the top.

5. Shell the egg, cut in half and place on top of the tuna.

6. Season with salt and freshly ground black pepper to serve.

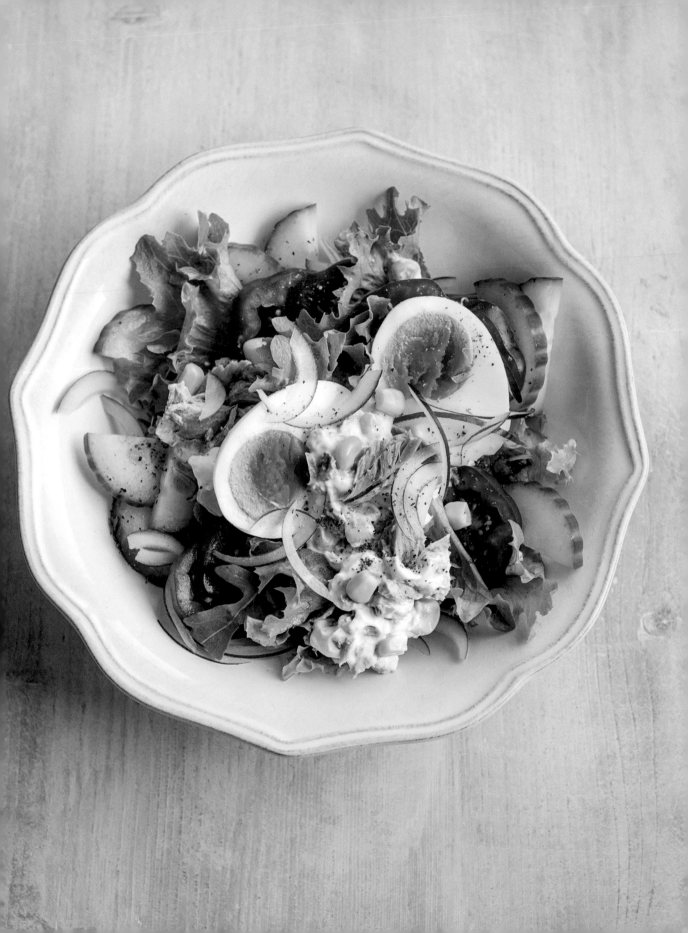

CALORIES: 270
Protein: 3.2g
Fats: 14.8g
Carbs: 31.5g

Vegan Nachos

SERVES 1

Meat eaters can make this higher protein by replacing the avocado with a small portion of chicken or lean beef mince.

1 small bag tortilla chips (approx. 30g)
½ red onion, peeled and diced
½ jalapeño pepper, sliced
20g any vegan cheese, grated
½ small avocado
½ tsp dried chilli flakes
1 tbsp fresh lime juice
1 tbsp salsa (homemade see page 180 or shop-bought)

1. Preheat the oven to 230°C/Fan 210°C.

2. Empty the tortilla chips into the centre of a baking tray and scatter over the onion and jalapeño.

3. Sprinkle the vegan cheese on top of the nachos and bake for 5 minutes, until the cheese starts to melt.

4. Meanwhile, mash the avocado with the chilli flakes and lime juice in a small bowl.

5. Remove the nachos from the oven, top with the avocado and salsa, season with salt and freshly ground black pepper and serve.

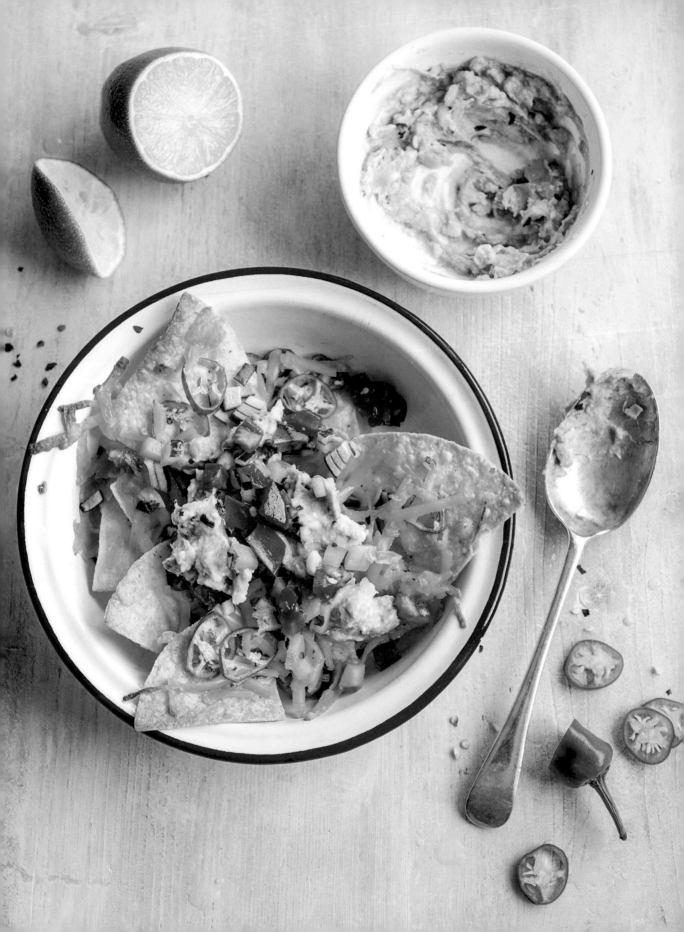

CALORIES: 236
Protein: 31.2g
Fats: 2.8g
Carbs: 20.3g

Greek Cottage Cheese

SERVES 1

I never liked cottage cheese because I kept trying it with fruit. When I tried it as a savoury snack, I was hooked! This tastes great eaten straight out of the mixing bowl but also works really well served in lettuce cups.

1 small tub fat-free cottage
   cheese (approx. 300g)
1 large handful black olives,
   sliced
½ small cucumber, diced
½ small tomato, diced
½ small red onion, peeled
   and diced
fresh thyme, oregano
   or parsley (optional)

1. Tip the cottage cheese into a small bowl and add the olives, cucumber, tomato, onion and herbs, if using. Mix well.

2. Season with salt and freshly ground pepper and serve.

COOK'S TIP

People are often surprised at the carb content of yoghurts and cheeses – don't forget that lactose is a carbohydrate!

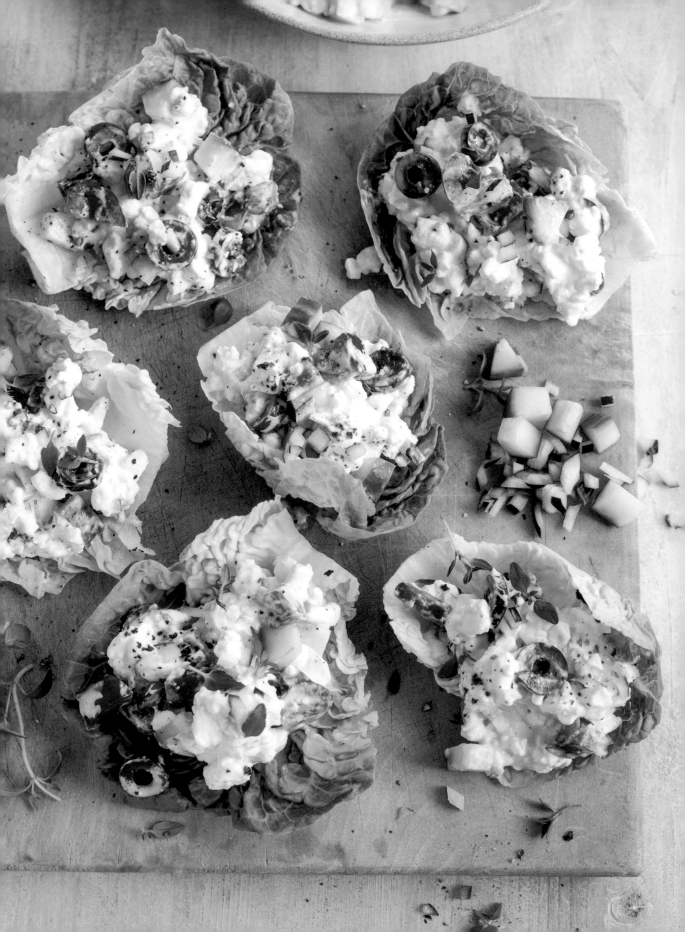

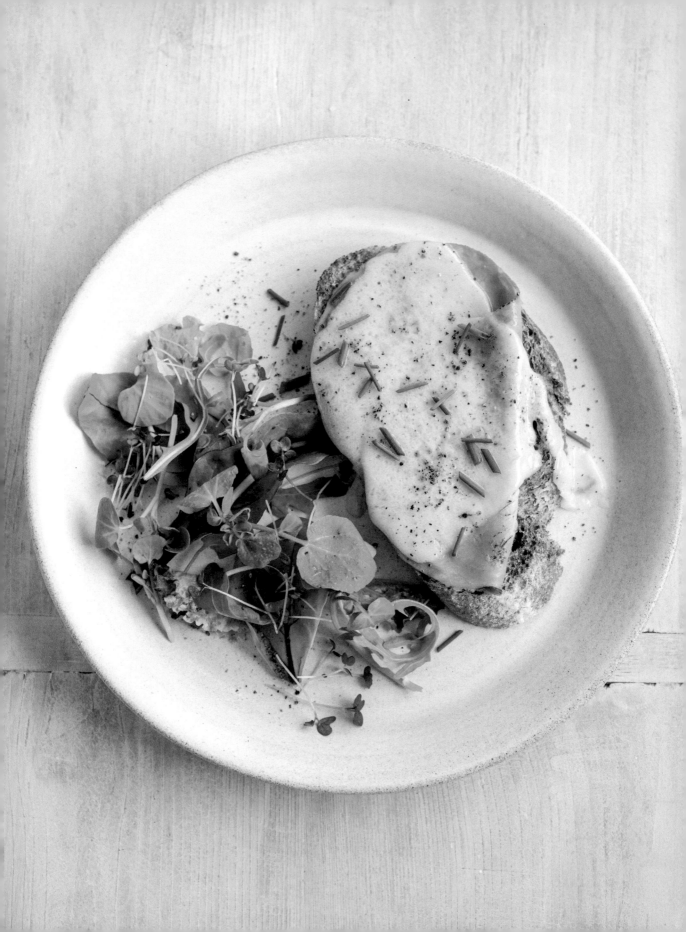

CALORIES: 265
Protein: 13.6g
Fats: 13.4g
Carbs: 22g

Quick and Simple Croque Monsieur

SERVES 1

Paprika works REALLY well on melted cheese, but chives are also great with this.

1 slice bread
   (typically 40–50g)
1 tsp salted butter
1 slice leam ham
1 slice mature Cheddar
   (approx. 20g)
1 tbsp chopped fresh
   chives (optional)
pinch paprika (optional)

1. Preheat the grill to high.

2. Butter the bread and place the ham on top. Lay the cheese on top of the ham and place under the grill for 5–10 minutes, until the cheese is bubbling.

3. Remove from the heat, sprinkle with the chives and paprika and serve with a side salad to get your micronutrients in!

This recipe is easily adapted for vegetarians by using Quorn slices instead of ham.

CALORIES: 290
Protein: 7.1g
Fats: 19.8g
Carbs: 27.2g

Spicy Nuts

SERVES 1

The ingredients, method, calories and macros are all for 1 serving. However, if you track, I advise that you cook these in bulk and simply divvy them up as 2 large handfuls per serving.

2 large handfuls mixed nuts
1 tbsp runny honey
½ tsp paprika
½ tsp chilli powder
½ tsp dried rosemary

This recipe is easily adapted for vegans by swapping the honey for maple syrup.

You could use fresh rosemary instead of dried. Add 1 teaspoon of finely chopped rosemary needles with the other ingredients in step 2.

1. Preheat the oven to 180°C/Fan 160°C.

2. Place all the ingredients except the rosemary in a bowl and mix together well.

3. Scatter them across a baking sheet and bake in the oven for 10–15 minutes until golden brown.

4. Remove from the oven and sprinkle over the rosemary.

5. Serve warm, seasoned with a touch of salt and freshly ground black pepper.

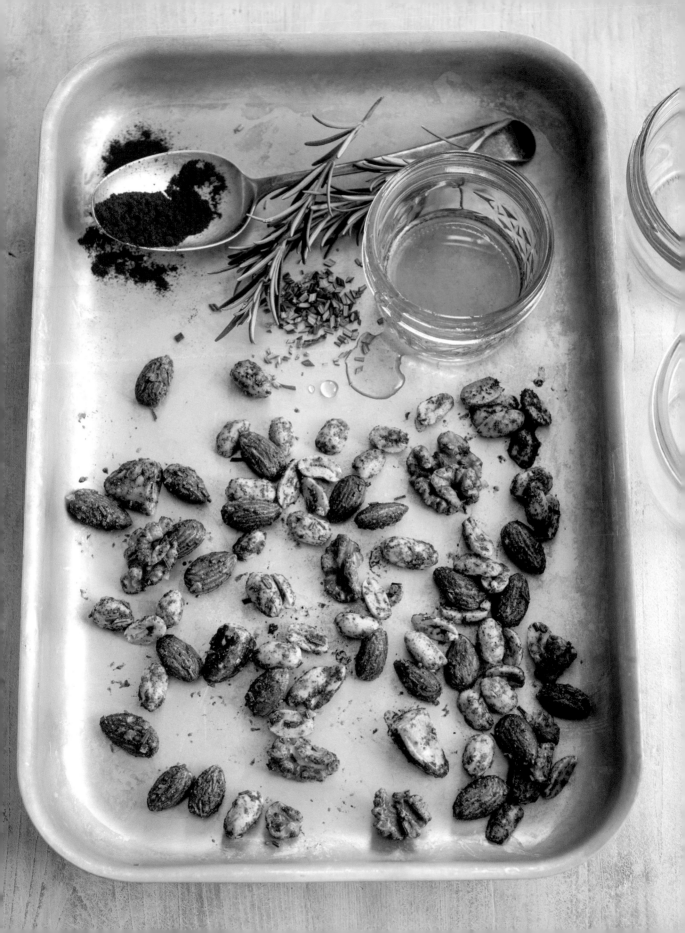

CALORIES: 266
Protein: 35.7g
Fats: 8.7g
Carbs: 10.2g

Chicken Satay Skewers

SERVES 1

This is a great snack for those of you with high protein dietary goals.

4 wooden skewers
1 chicken breast (typically
    125–150g), sliced into
    4 long strips
1 tbsp soy sauce (any)
1 tbsp fresh lemon juice
1 level tbsp crunchy peanut
    butter (homemade see
    page 183 or shop-bought)
1 tbsp hot sauce (any)
1 tsp runny honey
1 tsp chopped, crushed
    or puréed garlic
½ tsp ground ginger

1. Preheat the grill to medium and soak the wooden skewers in cold water.

2. Place the chicken in a large mixing bowl and add all the remaining ingredients. Mix well.

3. Thread the chicken strips through the skewers and place on a baking tray.

4. Grill the chicken skewers for 4–5 minutes on each side and serve!

COOK'S TIP

This recipe works really well if you leave the chicken to marinate in the fridge for a few hours.

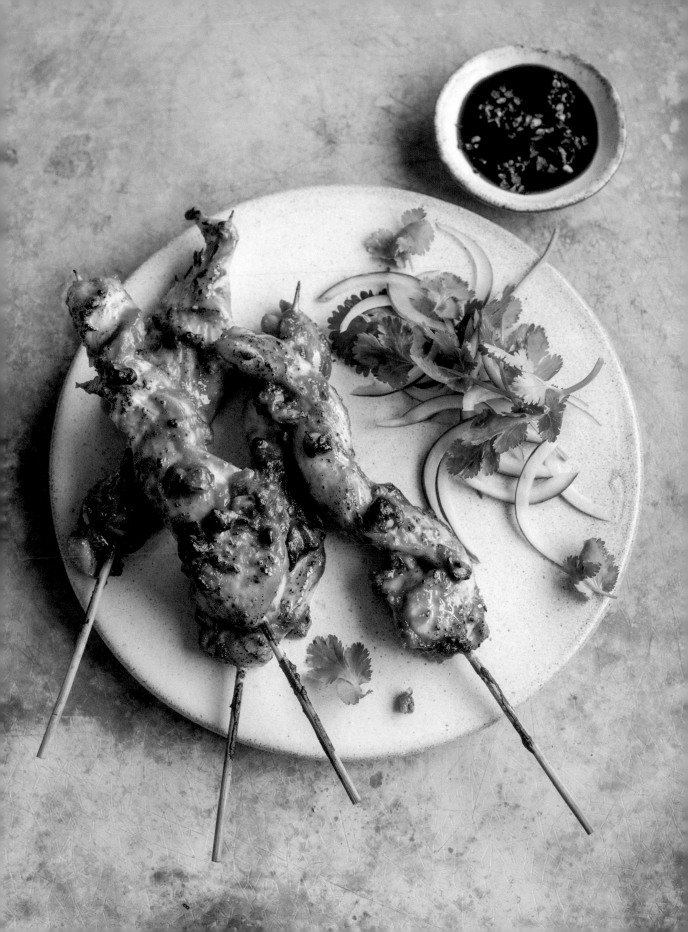

CALORIES: 242
Protein: 13.6g
Fats: 15g
Carbs: 8.1g

Garlic Roasted Broccoli and Tahini Drizzle

SERVES 1

Snacking on veg like this is a great idea when you're in a fat-loss phase. The calories are low, the fibre is high, and you will feel a lot more satiated than you would from eating a protein bar.

1 small head broccoli,
    broken into florets
1 tsp olive oil
3–4 garlic cloves, peeled
    and sliced
1 level tbsp light tahini
squeeze fresh lemon juice

COOK'S TIP

If you have a muscle-building goal, you can easily increase the calories by adding strips of pitta or torn flatbread to the broccoli, serving it with hummus or baba ganoush, or even by using this dish as a side to a lemon- and herb-marinated chicken breast.

1. Preheat the oven to 220°C/Fan 200°C.

2. Scatter the florets across a baking tray and drizzle with the olive oil. Season well with salt and freshly ground black pepper and roast in the oven for 10 minutes.

3. Remove from the oven, add the garlic and toss everything together. Return to the oven for a further 10 minutes, until the broccoli florets are tender and crispy.

4. Meanwhile, mix the tahini with the lemon juice and 1 tablespoon of water. Drizzle this over the broccoli, check the seasoning and serve.

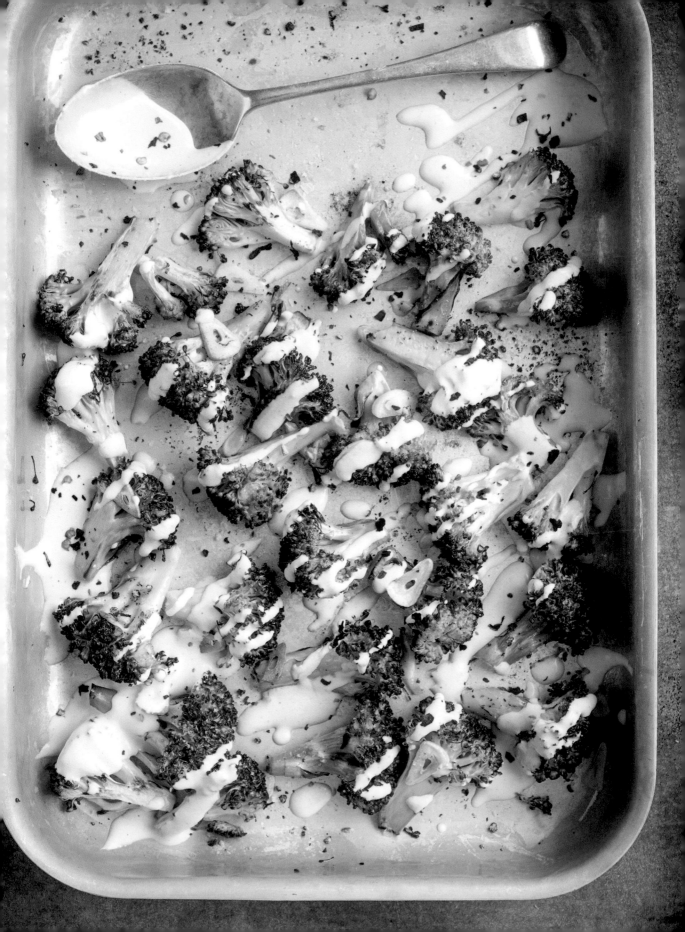

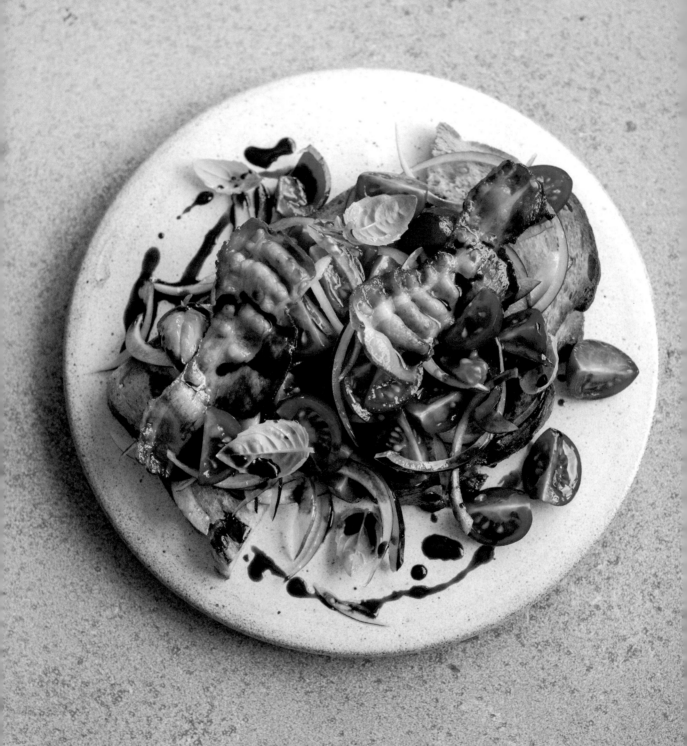

Pancetta Bruschetta

SERVES 1

Quick, easy and indulgent. I LOVE this recipe.

1 large handful cherry
   tomatoes, halved or
   quartered
½ small red onion, peeled
   and thinly sliced
2 tsp olive oil
2 slices pancetta
1 thick slice sourdough
   bread (typically 40–50g)
1 tbsp balsamic vinegar
   (any)
5–6 small fresh basil leaves

This recipe is easily
adapted for both
vegetarians and vegans
by removing or replacing
the pancetta with vegan
bacon, or any veg of
your choice.

1. Mix the cherry tomatoes and red onion together in a small bowl with 1 teaspoon of the olive oil. Season with salt and freshly ground black pepper.

2. Heat the remaining olive oil in a small non-stick frying pan over a high heat. When the oil starts to spit, add the pancetta and fry for 10 seconds on one side, then turn over.

3. As the second side cooks, place the sourdough in the pan alongside and let it soak up the olive oil.

4. When the pancetta is crispy and the sourdough has started to toast, remove both from the pan and place the pancetta on top of the bread.

5. Spoon the tomatoes over the top, drizzle with the balsamic vinegar and sprinkle with the basil. Check the seasoning and serve.

CALORIES: 299
Protein: 18.6g
Fats: 13.2g
Carbs: 28.4g

CALORIES: 283
Protein: 21.4g
Fats: 6.5g
Carbs: 37.8g

Oreo Milkshake

SERVES 1

Yes, you CAN have the odd treat and still be low calorie AND healthy!

1 scoop protein powder
300ml unsweetened nut milk (any)
3 Oreo cookies, crushed
5 ice cubes

1. Place the ingredients in a blender and whizz until you reach the desired consistency.

2. Pour into a glass to serve.

Beetroot and Berry Smoothie

SERVES 1

Healthy, high protein and a good energy booster!

1 large raw beetroot, peeled and
    chopped
1 large handful strawberries
1 large handful blueberries
1 large handful raspberries
1 small pot 0% Greek (or soy) yoghurt
    (approx. 170g)
300ml unsweetened nut milk
ice (if preferred)

1. Place the ingredients in a blender and whizz until you reach the desired consistency.

2. Pour into a glass to serve.

This recipe is easily adapted for vegans by using soy yoghurt instead of Greek.

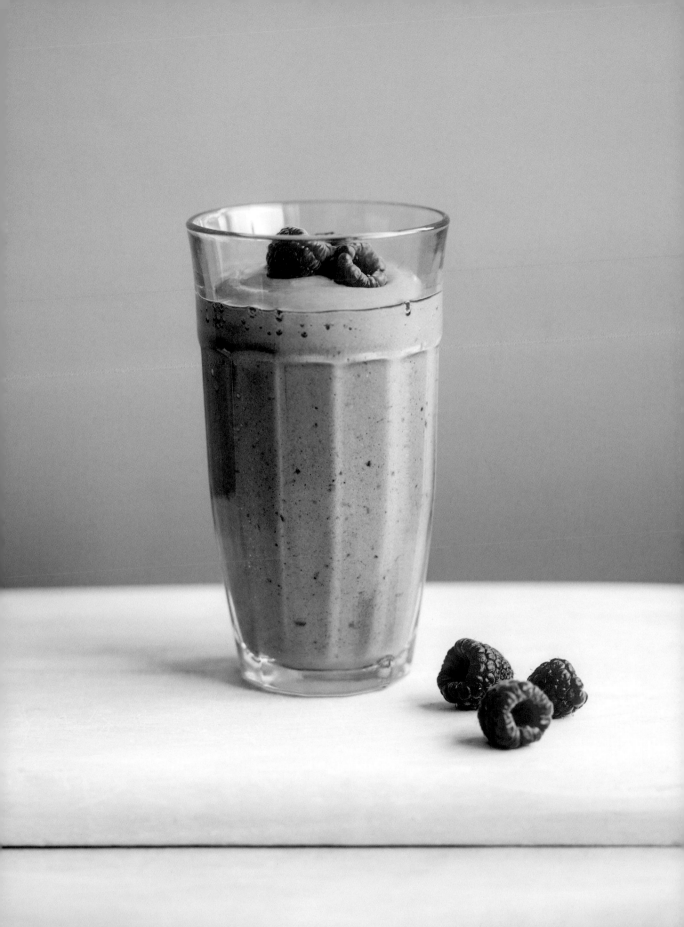

CALORIES: 139
Protein: 19.3g
Fats: 3.2g
Carbs: 9.3g

Victoria Sponge Protein Cake

SERVES 1

There's a nut butter version of this in my second book, *The Fat-loss Blitz*, and a chocolate version in my third, *Transform Your Body With Weights* – this time I'm going British!

1 scoop protein powder
dash unsweetened nut milk
    (any)
1 large handful
    strawberries, halved
1 heaped tbsp 0% Greek
    (or soy) yoghurt
½ tsp stevia (optional)

This recipe is easily adapted for vegans by using soy yoghurt instead of Greek. You can use any protein powder but I find that vanilla tastes best here.

1. Scoop the protein powder into a bowl or Tupperware. Stir in the milk to make a THICK batter (goopy, not runny) – you may need as much as 100ml milk, depending on your protein powder.

2. Smush the strawberries gently between your finger tips and stir half of them into the batter. Microwave for 2–3 minutes on high.

3. Meanwhile, stir the remaining strawberries into the Greek yoghurt.

4. Remove the cake from the microwave, spoon the yoghurt on top, sprinkle with the stevia, if using, and serve.

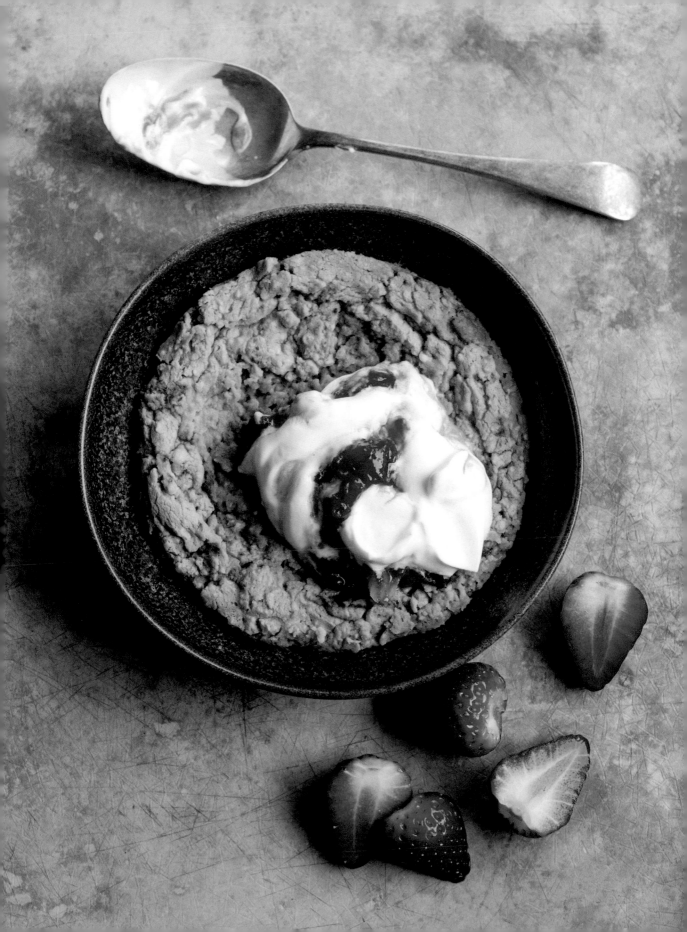

CALORIES: 299
Protein: 21.7g
Fats: 10.9g
Carbs: 33.2g

Protein Ice Cream

SERVES 1

A quick, sweet, indulgent snack!

1 small-medium banana,
    peeled, sliced then frozen
1 scoop protein powder
approx. 100ml
    unsweetened nut milk
    (any)
1 level tbsp chopped
    almonds
½ tsp stevia to sweeten

1. Add all ingredients to a blender and whizz for 1–2 minutes (stopping once or twice to scrape down the sides if necessary).

2. Spoon into a small bowl and serve.

A good pro tip is to cut up and freeze bananas en masse so you can make ice cream or milkshakes whenever your sweeet tooth strikes.

Peanut Butter Popcorn

SERVES 1

This is a great LOW-calorie, HIGH-energy snack!

1 tsp salted butter
1 large handful popcorn
   kernels
1 level tbsp smooth peanut
   butter (homemade see
   page 183 or shop-bought)
½ tsp stevia

This recipe is easily
adapted for vegans
by using coconut oil
instead of butter.

1. Melt the butter in a large saucepan over a medium heat then add the popcorn kernels. Cover the pan with a lid and shake the pan continuously to ensure the kernels coat in the butter and the popcorn doesn't catch. Cook for approximately 4 minutes, or until the popping stops. Remove from the heat and empty into a large bowl.

2. Meanwhile, spoon the nut butter into a small cup and microwave on high for 30 seconds.

3. Drizzle the nut butter over the popcorn, sprinkle with the stevia and serve.

CALORIES: 215
Protein: 3g
Fats: 8.4g
Carbs: 30.7g

Low-cal S'mores

SERVES 1

A perfect low-calorie, high-carb sweet treat!

2 large marshmallows
2 large, plain rice cakes
2 squares dark chocolate
(the darker the better)

COOK'S TIP

You could also bake these in the oven. Follow the steps and timings but bake in an oven preheated to 220°C/Fan 200°C.

1. Preheat the grill to high.

2. Put a marshmallow on top of each rice cake and place under the grill for 2–3 minutes.

3. As the marshmallows begin to melt, press a square of dark chocolate into each of them and continue to grill for a further 1–2 minutes, until the chocolate is partly melted.

4. Remove from the grill and serve.

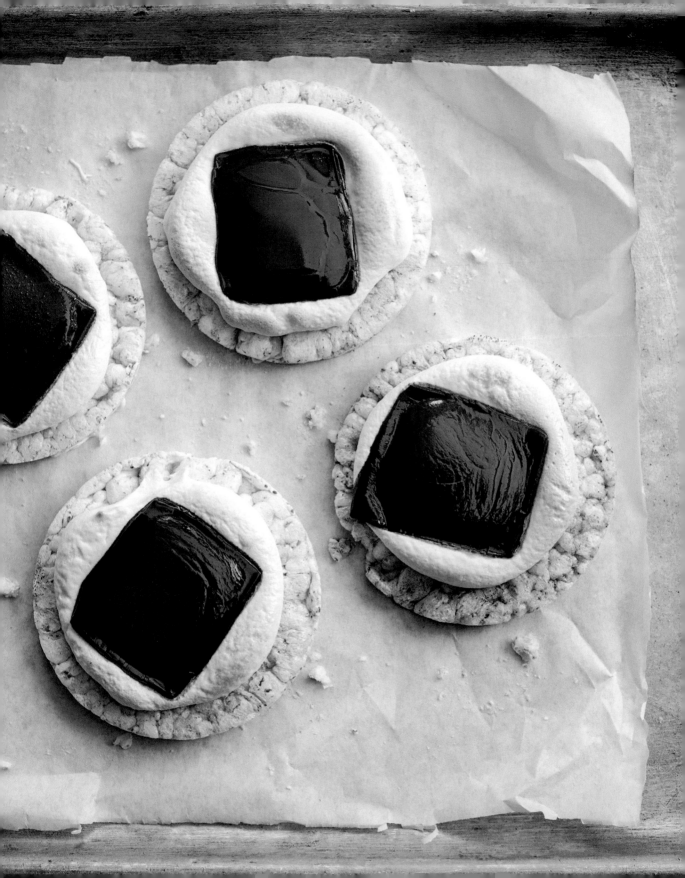

CALORIES: 210
Protein: 20.4g
Fats: 3.7g
Carbs: 23.3g

Blueberry Proats

SERVES 1

I've included proat recipes in all of my books – one peanut butter, one banana and one Nutella! Proats are a body builder staple for a reason – protein and carbs are exactly what you need both pre- and post-training, regardless of goals.

1 sachet / 1 handful oats
    (approx. 30g)
1 scoop protein powder
1 large handful blueberries,
    halved
pinch ground cinnamon
    (optional)

COOK'S
TIP

You can use any protein powder but I find that strawberry or vanilla taste best here.

1. Boil the kettle.

2. Empty the oats and protein powder into a bowl and pour boiling water into the bowl, stirring as you do. I like my proats quite thick, but feel free to keep adding water until the mixture reaches your desired consistency (you'll need approximately 200ml).

3. Scatter the berries on top and sprinkle with the cinnamon, if using, to serve.

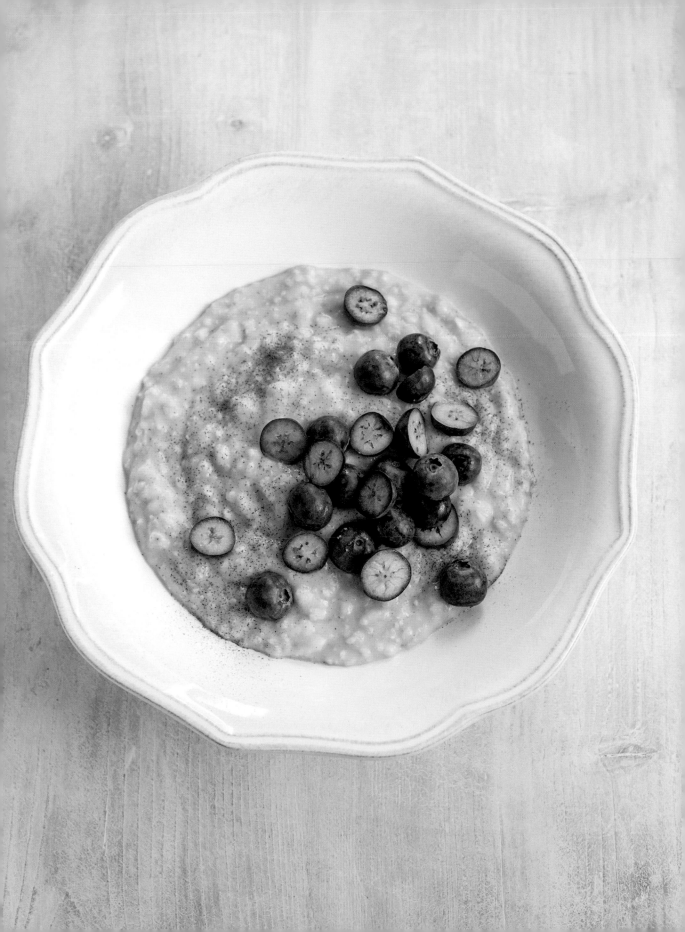

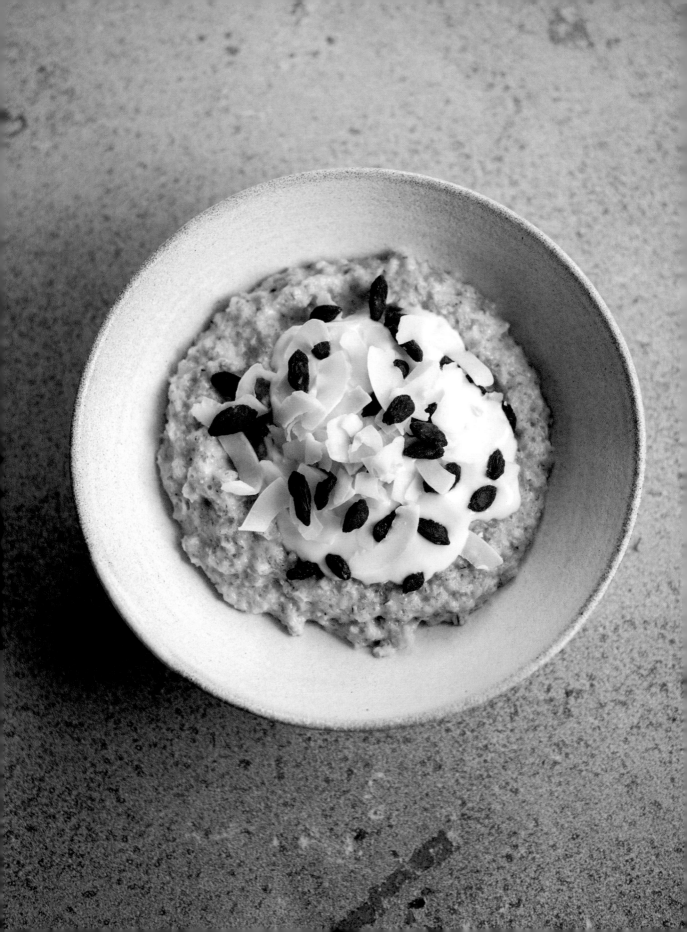

CALORIES: 262
Protein: 5.6g
Fats: 17.1g
Carbs: 18.1g

Creamy Coconut Porridge

SERVES 1

This is a great fix for a rumbly tummy on a cold day.

1 sachet / 1 handful oats (approx. 30g)
approx. 200ml unsweetened coconut milk
2 heaped tbsp coconut yoghurt
1 tbsp desiccated coconut or 2 tbsp coconut flakes
½ tsp stevia
1 tbsp goji berries (optional)

1. If you are cooking in a microwave, stir the oats and milk together in a bowl and cook on high for 2–3 minutes. Alternatively, stir the oats and milk in a small saucepan over a medium heat for 2–3 minutes.

2. Remove from the heat and stir in 1 tablespoon of the yoghurt.

3. Dollop the second tablespoon of yoghurt on top of the porridge, sprinkle over the coconut, stevia and goji berries, if using, and serve.

CALORIES: 288
Protein: 14.5g
Fats: 13.2g
Carbs: 27g

Crunchy French Toast

SERVES 1

This is one of my husband's favourites. It's quick and easy to make, is macro friendly and will hit your sweet tooth!

1 large egg (or 2 small)
½ tsp stevia (optional)
1 slice bread (typically 40–50g)
1 level tbsp crunchy nut butter (homemade see page 183 or shop-bought)
1 tsp maple syrup

Double up on this for a great muscle-building / performance breakfast.

1. Whisk the egg(s) in a bowl and sprinkle in the stevia, if using.

2. Place the bread in the egg mixture and leave it to soak.

3. Place a non-stick frying pan over a high heat. Lay the bread in the centre of the pan and cook for 1–2 minutes. Turn it over, reduce the heat to medium and cook for another few minutes.

4. Once the toast is an even, golden brown, plate it up and spoon the nut butter over the top – it will melt a little. Drizzle with the maple syrup and serve!

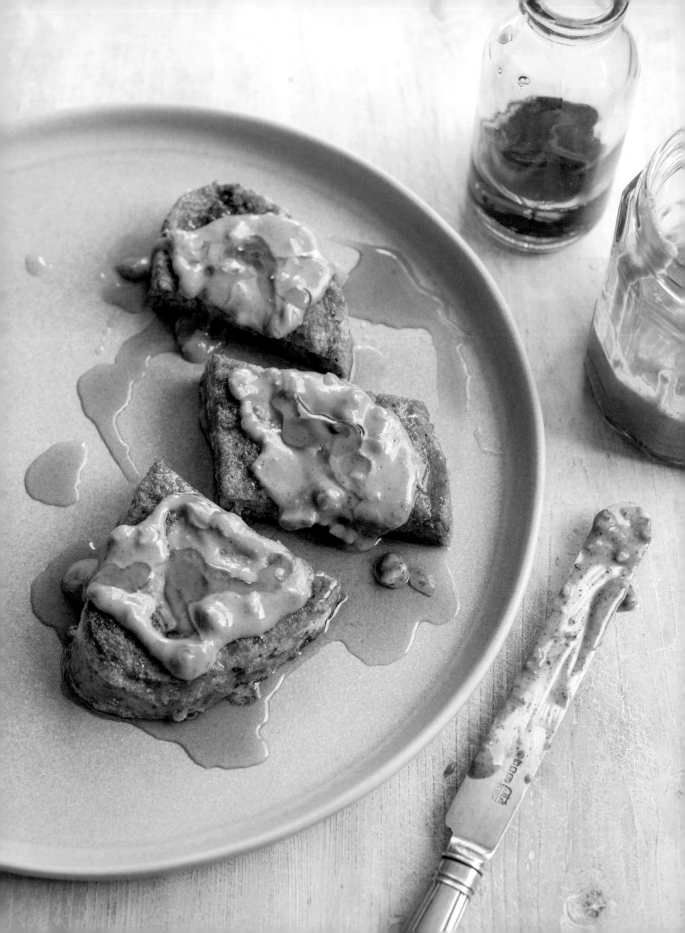

CALORIES: 260
Protein: 6.5g
Fats: 7.3g
Carbs: 41.8g

3 Ingredient Rice Krispie Treats

SERVES 1

I've edited this to be 1 serving for 1 person, making it far easier for both trackers and non-trackers to keep tabs on their food intake. I started making these as pre-workout energy snacks a few months ago and when I'm in a fat-loss phase, it is honestly my favourite time of day!

1 large handful / small
   variety packet Rice
   Krispies (approx. 30g)
1 level tbsp smooth nut
   butter (homemade see
   page 183 or shop-bought)
1 tbsp maple syrup

COOK'S
TIP

Remember you'll need a small dish in order for these to harden as one single serving. Alternatively, increase the quantities and make a bigger slab, then divide into multiple portions.

1. Tip the Rice Krispies into a small bowl.

2. Mix the nut butter and syrup together in a small cup and microwave on high for 30 seconds. Once the nut butter and syrup have melted together, immediately spoon over the Rice Krispies. Stir all three ingredients together well, making sure you coat the cereal completely.

3. Push the mixture down into the bottom of the bowl using the back of a spoon so that it is compact, or press into two small tart tins. Place the bowl / tins in the freezer for 10–15 minutes then remove.

4. Slide a knife around the edges of the Rice Krispie treat – it should be cold enough and compact enough to lift right out.

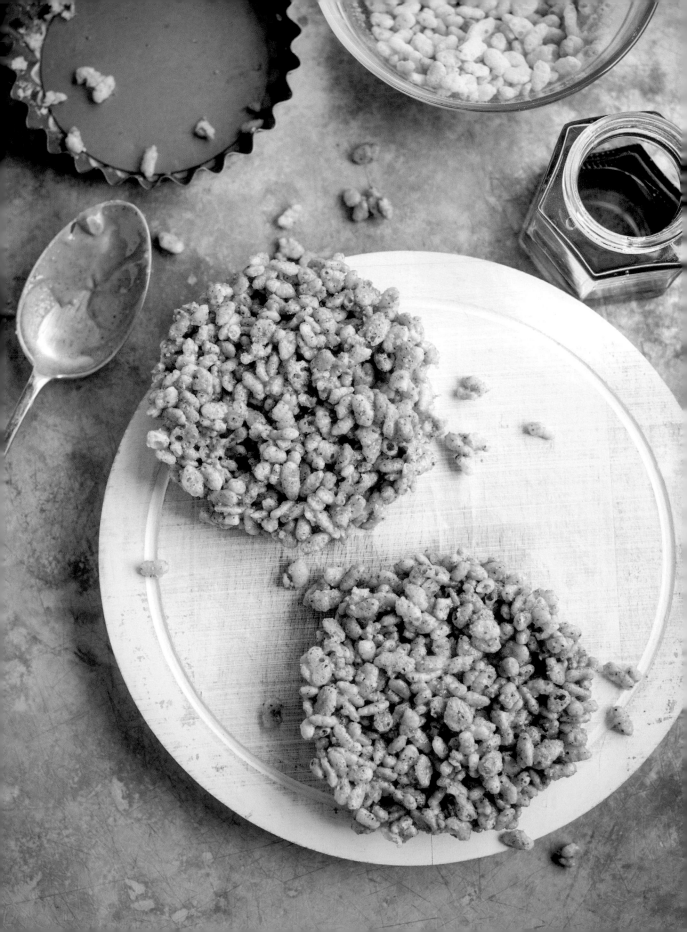

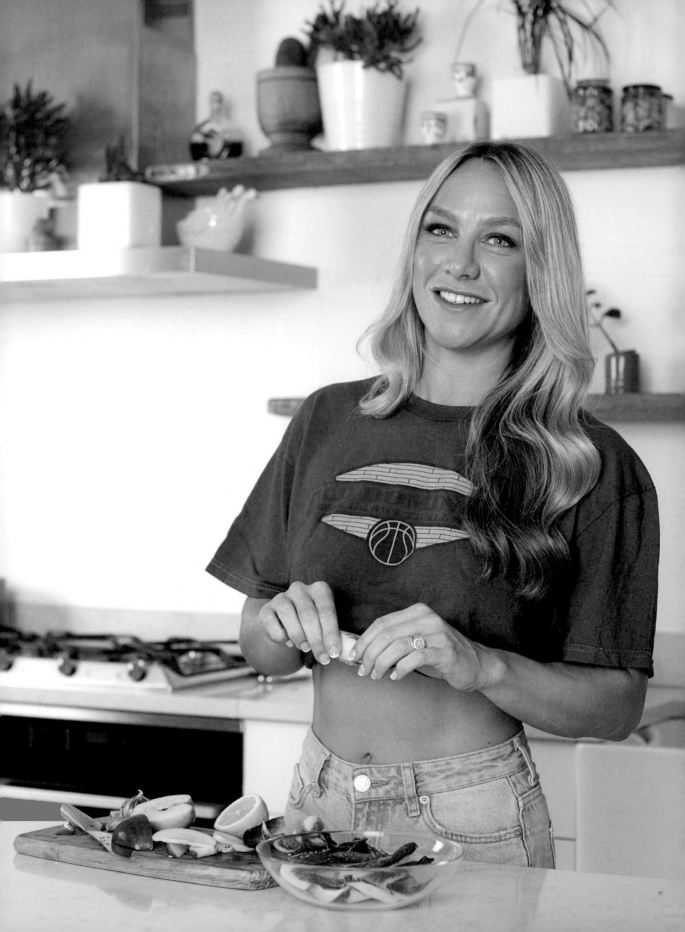

EXTRAS

●○○

A few extra recipes that are
good to have up your sleeve.

PER QUANTITY
CALORIES: 120
Protein: 4.4g
Fats: 0.8g
Carbs: 28.1g

PER TABLESPOON
CALORIES: 4
Protein: 0.2g
Fats: 0.01g
Carbs: 0.35g

Homemade Salsa

MAKES 450G

Store-bought or homemade, salsa is a great low-calorie dip for dieters!

3 large tomatoes, chopped
½ yellow pepper, finely diced
½ red onion, peeled and finely diced
½ packet fresh coriander (approx. 12g), finely chopped
zest and juice of ½ lime
1 tbsp sweet chilli sauce

1. Place a sieve over a large bowl and strain the tomatoes to remove some of the liquid.

2. Place the strained tomatoes in another bowl with the remaining ingredients, season with salt and freshly ground black pepper and mix well.

COOK'S TIP

This will make four large portions – if you aren't going to eat it all at once, you can freeze portions for another day. You could use 1 × 400g tin chopped tomatoes to make this salsa if you don't have fresh tomatoes.

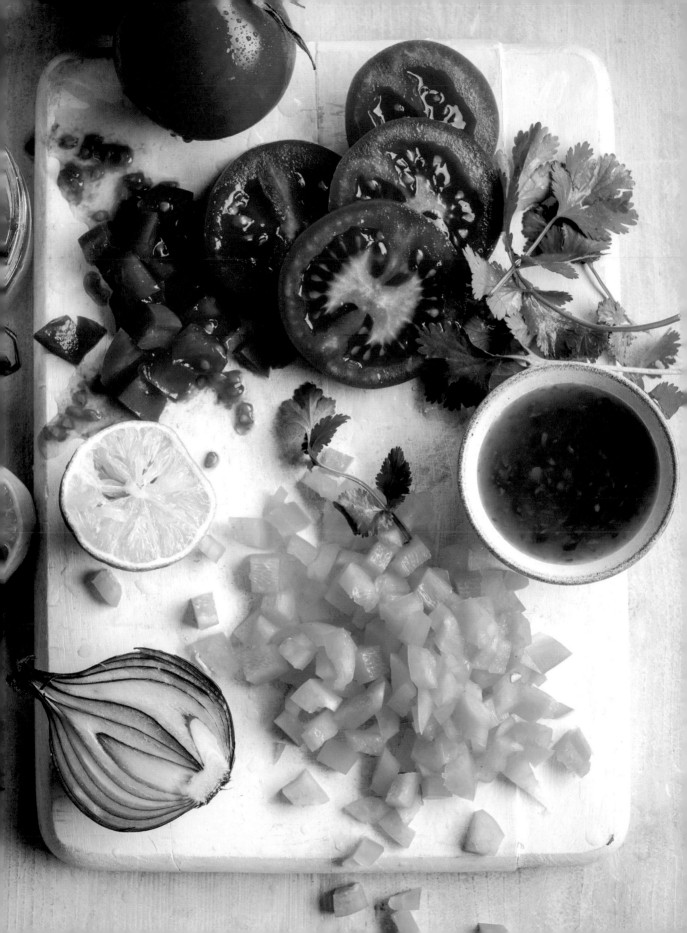

PER QUANTITY
CALORIES: 642
Protein: 39.7g
Fats: 2.3g
Carbs: 175.3g

PER 200G PORTION
CALORIES: 128
Protein: 7.9g
Fats: 0.5g
Carbs: 35g

Homemade Baked Beans

MAKES 5 PORTIONS

This recipe will make roughly five portions. Try them with a jacket potato and cheese (see page 100).

500g passata
½ onion (any), peeled
   and finely chopped
40g brown sugar or
   2 tbsp stevia
3 tbsp reduced salt and
   sugar ketchup
1 tbsp white wine vinegar
1 tsp smoked paprika
   (optional)
dash vegan Worcestershire
   sauce
1 × 400g tin pinto beans,
   drained and rinsed
1 × 400g tin haricot beans,
   drained and rinsed

1. Place all the ingredients in a saucepan over a medium heat. Season with salt and freshly ground black pepper and mix well.

2. Bring to a simmer and cook uncovered for 10 minutes.

COOK'S TIP

If you use stevia instead of sugar when you make these beans, the total calorie count is reduced from 642 to 490. The carb count is also reduced from 175.3g to 136.3g.

PER QUANTITY
CALORIES: 1737
Protein: 63.4g
Fats: 149.8g
Carbs: 64.6g

PER TABLESPOON
CALORIES: 87
Protein: 3.2g
Fats: 7.5g
Carbs: 3.2g

Homemade Nut Butter

MAKES 300G

For those keen cooks who like to make everything from scratch! The quantities here will give you roughly 20 level tablespoons of nut butter.

300g raw almonds (or any other raw nut – peanuts, pecans and hazelnuts are also good)
pinch sea salt

COOK'S TIP

Hazelnuts and peanuts have skins and it is better to remove them before you whizz. Just rub the roasted nuts with a tea towel.

1. Preheat the oven to 170°C/Fan 150°C.

2. Tip the nuts on to a baking tray and roast in the oven for 8–10 minutes.

3. Remove from the oven and place in a blender. Whizz for 3 minutes, then scrape down the sides and whizz again for another 3 minutes. Scrape down the sides and whizz for a final 3 minutes – the nut butter should be lovely and smooth. Season with the salt and stir well.

4. Transfer to a sterilised container and keep covered in the fridge for up to 1 month.

PER QUANTITY
CALORIES: 2846
Protein: 76.8g
Fats: 108.9g
Carbs: 396.8g

PER 100G PORTION
CALORIES: 355.8
Protein: 9.6g
Fats: 13.6g
Carbs: 49.6g

Homemade Granola

MAKES 8 PORTIONS

All granola packs a calorie punch so if you have a fat-loss goal, use sparingly. The macros look huge when you make a large portion like this but, remember, you'll only be using 100g or so at any one time.

100g runny honey
100g brown sugar
50ml sunflower oil
1 tsp vanilla extract
½ tsp salt
320g oats
75g sunflower seeds
75g pumpkin seeds
75g raw almonds

This recipe is easily adapted for vegans simply by swapping the honey for maple syrup.

1. Preheat the oven to 150°C/Fan 130°C.

2. Place the honey and sugar in a small saucepan over a gentle heat and melt together, stirring all the time.

3. Place all the other ingredients in a large bowl, then pour in the honey and sugar mixture. Mix well.

4. Tip on to a baking tray and spread out evenly. Cook in the oven for 30–40 minutes, stirring and turning the granola every 10 minutes.

5. Remove from the oven and leave to cool.

6. Tip into an airtight container and store for up to 3 months.

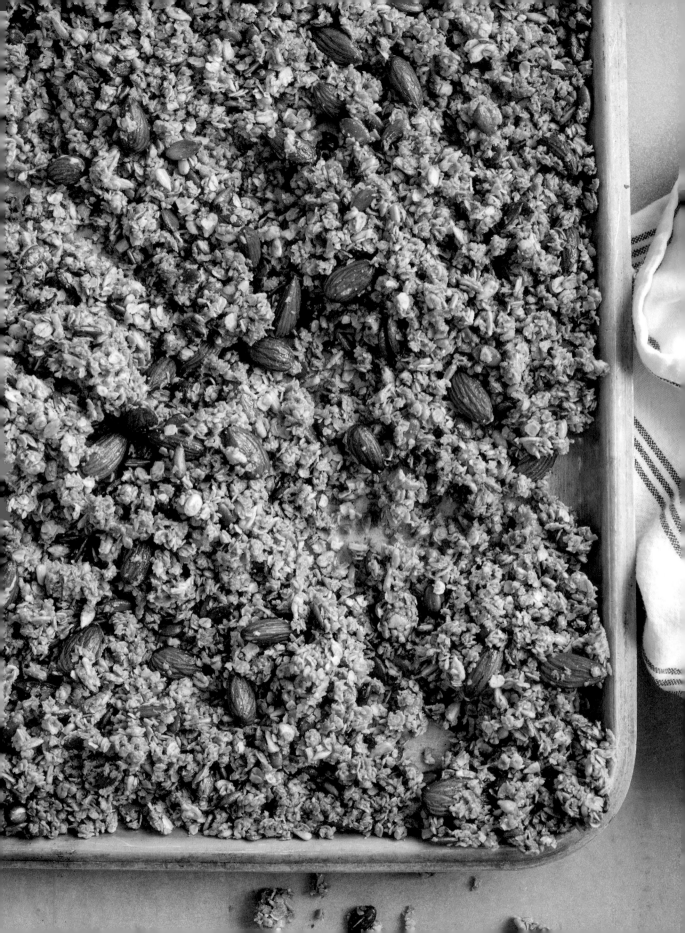

PER QUANTITY
CALORIES: 542
Protein: 10.4g
Fats: 41.3g
Carbs: 38.1g

PER 150G PORTION
CALORIES: 180
Protein: 3g
Fats: 14g
Carbs: 13g

Any Veg Coleslaw

MAKES 3 PORTIONS

You can swap the veg in this recipe for whatever you have in your fridge – so long as it's possible to grate it and eat it raw. Cabbage works well and hard fruit, like apples and pears, would too. This recipe will make approximately 450g coleslaw and provides three generous portions.

2 small raw beetroots (approx. 100g total weight), peeled
3 carrots, peeled
150g celeriac, peeled
½ small red onion, peeled and sliced (optional)
1 tbsp light mayonnaise
½ tsp Dijon mustard
1 tbsp cider vinegar
2 tbsp olive oil
pinch sugar or stevia
½ bunch fresh flat-leaf parsley (approx. 15g), roughly chopped
2 tbsp pumpkin seeds, toasted

1. Using a food processor or large grater, grate the beetroot, carrots and celeriac and tip into a large bowl. Stir in the red onion, if using.

2. Combine the mayonnaise, mustard, vinegar and oil in a small bowl or jug and whisk together well. Stir in the sugar or stevia and season with salt and freshly ground black pepper.

3. Pour this dressing over the grated veg and sprinkle with the parsley. Mix well to coat.

4. Sprinkle with the pumpkin seeds to serve.

This recipe is easily adapted for vegans simply by using vegan mayonaise.

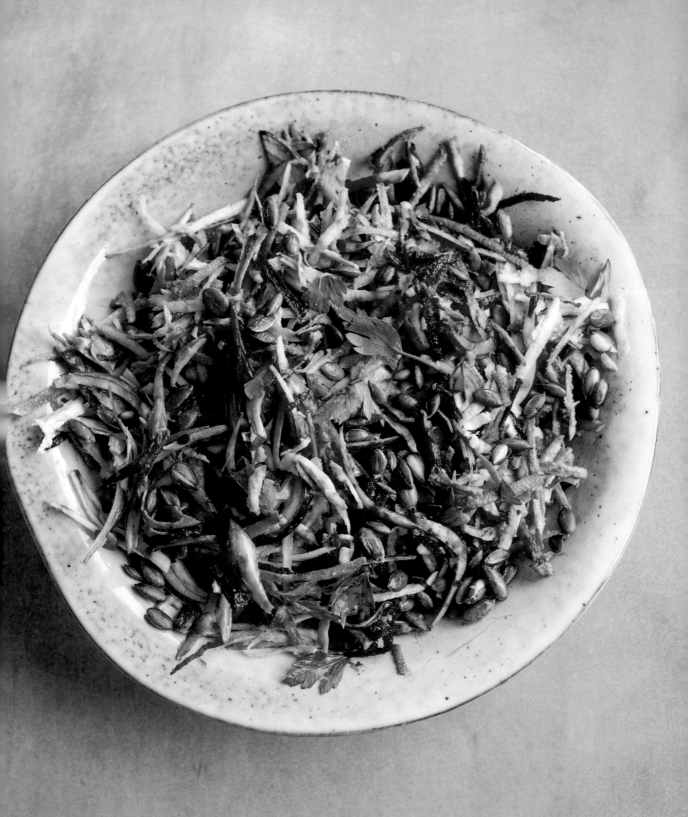

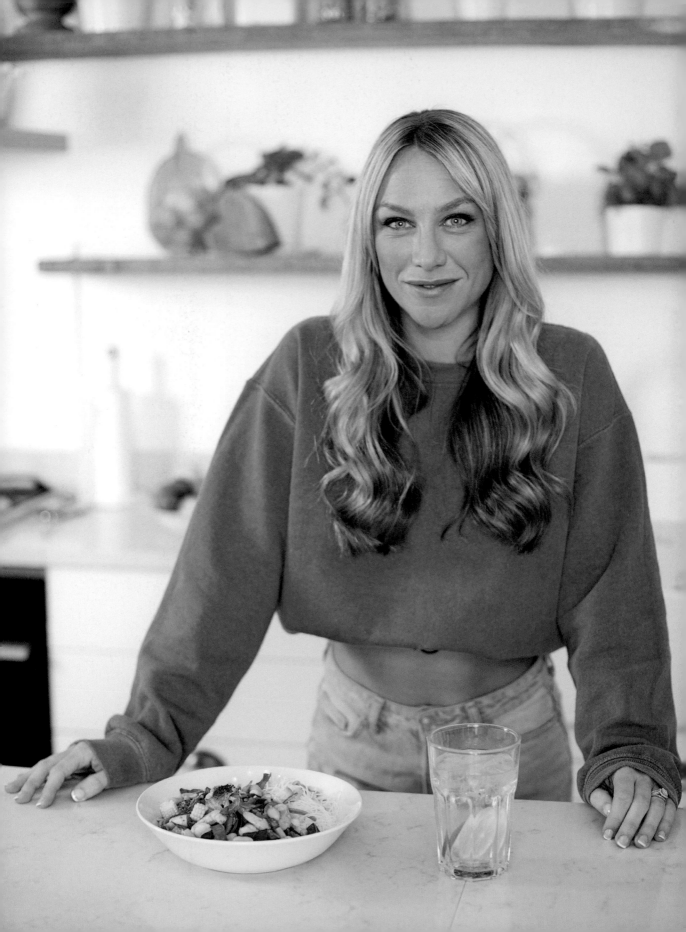

MEAL PLANS

○ ● ○

You do not have to follow these meal plans, they are just here to help give you some structure if you need it, or for reference as examples. They should give you a good idea of what to eat, when and how much your daily calorie intake should be (roughly), depending on your goal.

I've tried to structure them so they work easily with a Monday–Friday work week (whether prepping or eating on the go), and lazier Saturday–Sunday weekends.

Fat-loss Goals

In **A Quick Word on Calorie Intakes** I outlined exactly what a fat-loss diet needs (a calorie deficit). Without going through it all again, I'd like to highlight a few of the *key* points.

>> The universally recommended calorie intake for women is 2000kcals per day
>> 1lb is estimated to total about 3500kcals

So, for a woman to lose 1lb a week, the equation looks like this:

2000kcals per day x 7 = 14,000kcals per week (maintenance)
14,000kcals per week – 3500kcals (1lb) = 10,500kcals per week (weight loss)
10,500kcals per week / 7 = 1500kcals per day

This is called a 'standard' female calorie deficit.

PLEASE NOTE
These numbers are AVERAGES. I've had female clients achieve fantastic fat loss on 2000kcals per day, and I've had to drop clients down to 1200kcals to see results. Different heights, weights, ages, hormones, genetics and jobs all factor when determining what calories work best for the *individual*.

Also, our metabolisms (our body's ability to burn calories for energy) are ADAPTIVE, meaning the longer we eat in a deficit, the more our metabolic rate slows down to match our food intake.

As a result, the best way to implement a calorie deficit is to start with a higher calorie count and monitor your weekly results. If you aren't dropping weight, you aren't in a deficit yet, so reduce your intake.

Muscle-building and Performance Goals

Hypertrophy (muscle building) is achieved in the gym with the right weight-lifting plan, coupled with a high-calorie, high-protein and high-carbohydrate diet.

Performance is also a training goal that is fuelled via higher calories and macros.

>> In order for your body to perform at 100% and / or add mass (muscle), you need to FUEL and FEED it.

>> You do not need to OVEREAT and pile on the pounds by any means, but you DO need to expect a small amount of fat gain and focus more on your training and recovery than your aesthetic physique.

General Health and Fitness Goals

General health and fitness goals call for nutritious, well-balanced, calorie- and macro-aware meals.

>> Don't be overly concerned with how you look, focus more on how you feel. This is where good nutrition really comes into play...

PLEASE NOTE

>> Men with a fat-loss goal need to hit around 2000kcals per day, which will see them in a daily deficit of around 500kcals.

>> Men with a muscle-building and / or performance goal need to hit around 3000kcals per day, which will see them in a daily surplus of around 500kcals.

>> Men with a general health and fitness goal need to hit around 2500kcals per day, which will see them at a healthy maintenance intake.

>> You can follow the meal plans and make up the added calories however you like. I personally suggest swapping snacks for meals, which will pull your calories up and be very easy to implement, but you can add them whenever and however you please!

FAT-LOSS MEAL PLANS

Monday

BREAKFAST
Crunchy Banana Shake
Calories: 365

AM SNACK
Greek Cottage Cheese
Calories: 236

LUNCH
Torn Mozzarella and Chicken Salad
Calories: 326

PM SNACK
Spicy Nuts
Calories: 290

DINNER
Prawns, Shoots and Leaves
Calories: 395

TOTAL CALORIES: 1612

Tuesday

BREAKFAST
The Lean Greens Shake
Calories: 388

AM SNACK
Peanut Butter Popcorn
Calories: 237

LUNCH
The Healthy PB & J
Calories: 389

PM SNACK
Chicken Satay Skewers
Calories: 266

DINNER
Fillet Steak and Mushroom Medley
Calories: 323

TOTAL CALORIES: 1603

Wednesday

BREAKFAST
Peanut Choc Yog Pot
Calories: 364

AM SNACK
Beetroot and Berry Smoothie
Calories: 283

LUNCH
Club Flatbread
Calories: 396

PM SNACK
Cheesy Popcorn
Calories: 300

DINNER
Traybake Salmon and Fennel
Calories: 366

TOTAL CALORIES: 1709

Thursday

BREAKFAST
Spicy Overnight Oats
Calories: 395

AM SNACK
3 Ingredient Rice Krispie Treats
Calories: 260

LUNCH
Smoked Salmon Wraps
Calories: 360

PM SNACK
Garlic Roasted Broccoli and Tahini Drizzle
Calories: 242

DINNER
Fast Fried Rice
Calories: 393

TOTAL CALORIES: 1650

Friday

 BREAKFAST
Eton Morning Mess
Calories: 387

 AM SNACK
Oreo Milkshake
Calories: 299

 LUNCH
Torn Mozzarella and Chicken Salad
Calories: 326

 PM SNACK
Pancetta Bruschetta
Calories: 299

 DINNER
Fish, Chips and Crunchy Sprouts!
Calories: 421

TOTAL CALORIES: 1732

Saturday

 BREAKFAST
Mexican Omelette
Calories: 357

 AM SNACK
Protein Ice Cream
Calories: 299

 LUNCH
Mexican Bean and Brown Rice Bowl
Calories: 398

 PM SNACK
Low-cal S'mores
Calories: 215

 DINNER
Fillet Steak and Mushroom Medley
Calories: 323

TOTAL CALORIES: 1592

Sunday

 BREAKFAST
Lean Beans On Toast
Calories: 361

 AM SNACK
Crunchy French Toast
Calories: 288

 LUNCH
Fish, Chips and Crunchy Sprouts!
Calories: 421

 PM SNACK
Victoria Sponge Protein Cake
Calories: 139

 DINNER
Curried Chicken and Broccoli Rice
Calories: 335

TOTAL CALORIES: 1544

If you work 9–5, it's a good idea to have breakfasts like shakes, overnight oats or yoghurt pots pre-prepared Monday to Friday.

While meal prepping your lunches will also help you stay on track, most supermarkets, cafés and even fast food chains offer nutritious and calorie-conscious salads and snacks nowadays.

MUSCLE-BUILDING / PERFORMANCE MEAL PLAN

Monday

  BREAKFAST
Protein Ice Cream Shake
Calories: 674

  AM SNACK
Egg White Omelette
Calories: 177

 LUNCH
Salad Niçoise with a Kick
Calories: 797

  PM SNACK
Blueberry Proats
Calories: 210

 DINNER
Creamy Chicken and Mushroom Rice
Calories: 818

TOTAL CALORIES: 2676

Tuesday

 BREAKFAST
Bacon Avocado Toastie
Calories: 672

  AM SNACK
Creamy Coconut Porridge
Calories: 262

 LUNCH
Grilled Salmon Wholegrain Salad
Calories: 887

 PM SNACK
Quick and Simple Croque Monsieur
Calories: 265

  DINNER
Protein Traybake
Calories: 594

TOTAL CALORIES: 2680

Wednesday

  BREAKFAST
Melt-in-the-Middle Protein Oats
Calories: 499

  AM SNACK
Peanut Butter Popcorn
Calories: 237

 LUNCH
My Steak Baguette
Calories: 635

 PM SNACK
Tuna Salad
Calories: 249

 DINNER
Chilli Prawn Pasta
Calories: 696

TOTAL CALORIES: 2316

Thursday

 BREAKFAST
My New York Bagel with a Twist
Calories: 524

  AM SNACK
Beetroot and Berry Smoothie
Calories: 283

  LUNCH
High Protein Quesadilla
Calories: 722

  PM SNACK
Greek Cottage Cheese
Calories: 236

  DINNER
Jacket Potato with Cheese and Beans
Calories: 632

TOTAL CALORIES: 2397

Friday

 BREAKFAST
Burrito to Go!
Calories: 547

 AM SNACK
3 Ingredient Rice Krispie Treats
Calories: 260

 LUNCH
Tofu Hummus Wraps
Calories: 609

 PM SNACK
Spicy Nuts
Calories: 290

 DINNER
Creamy Chicken and Mushroom Rice
Calories: 818

TOTAL CALORIES: 2524

Saturday

 BREAKFAST
American Toast
Calories: 704

 AM SNACK
Oreo Milkshake
Calories: 299

 LUNCH
Salad Niçoise with a Kick
Calories: 797

 PM SNACK
Vegan Nachos
Calories: 270

 DINNER
Quick and Simple Carbonara
Calories: 714

TOTAL CALORIES: 2784

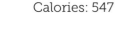

Sunday

  BREAKFAST
Flourless Honey Pancakes
Calories: 631

 AM SNACK
Low-cal S'mores
Calories: 215

 LUNCH
Vegan Sunday Roast
Calories: 573

 PM SNACK
Chicken Satay Skewers
Calories: 266

  DINNER
Protein Traybake
Calories: 594

TOTAL CALORIES: 2279

Obviously, having a target of 2000–3000kcals a day means that eating on the go while achieving your goals becomes a lot easier to do. However, remember that good-quality, nutrient-dense foods DO still matter when you have a muscle-building and / or performance goal. It's particularly important to get enough protein. For this reason, try to prep your own food as often as you can.

GENERAL HEALTH AND FITNESS MEAL PLAN

Monday

BREAKFAST
Antioxidant Protein Porridge
Calories: 404

———

AM SNACK
Protein Ice Cream
Calories: 299

———

LUNCH
Herby Lemon Chicken Salad
Calories: 499

———

PM SNACK
Garlic Roasted Broccoli
and Tahini Drizzle
Calories: 242

———

DINNER
Black Bean Burrito
Calories: 542

———

TOTAL CALORIES: 1986

Tuesday

BREAKFAST
Vit C Smoothie
Calories: 489

———

AM SNACK
3 Ingredient Rice Krispie Treats
Calories: 260

———

LUNCH
Vegan Pitta
Calories: 547

———

PM SNACK
Pancetta Bruschetta
Calories: 299

———

DINNER
Pork Fillet and Cheesy New Potatoes
Calories: 569

———

TOTAL CALORIES: 2164

Wednesday

  BREAKFAST
The Matcha Smoothie
Calories: 517

———

 AM SNACK
Low-cal S'mores
Calories: 215

———

 LUNCH
Spicy Chicken Salad
Calories: 444

———

  PM SNACK
Victoria Sponge Protein Cake
Calories: 139

———

 DINNER
Ratatouille Cod
Calories: 411

———

TOTAL CALORIES: 1726

Thursday

  BREAKFAST
Good Gut Grains
Calories: 471

———

  AM SNACK
Egg White Omelette
Calories: 177

———

 LUNCH
Tuna Pasta with an Upgrade!
Calories: 523

———

  PM SNACK
Vegan Nachos
Calories: 270

———

 DINNER
Sweet Potato, Cauliflower,
Squash and Chicken Traybake
Calories: 438

———

TOTAL CALORIES: 1879

Friday

BREAKFAST
Poached Eggs and Avocado on Toast
Calories: 476

AM SNACK
Blueberry Proats
Calories: 210

LUNCH
Herby Lemon Chicken Salad
Calories: 499

PM SNACK
Quick and Simple Croque Monsieur
Calories: 265

DINNER
Salmon Ramen
Calories: 604

TOTAL CALORIES: 2054

Saturday

BREAKFAST
Blueberry Protein Pancakes
Calories: 455

AM SNACK
Creamy Coconut Porridge
Calories: 262

LUNCH
Black Bean Burrito
Calories: 542

PM SNACK
Peanut Butter Popcorn
Calories: 237

DINNER
Spicy Chicken Sausage Pasta
Calories: 488

TOTAL CALORIES: 1984

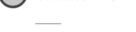

Sunday

 BREAKFAST
The Nutrient Omelette
Calories: 405

 AM SNACK
Beetroot and Berry Smoothie
Calories: 283

 LUNCH
Vegan Pitta
Calories: 547

 PM SNACK
Greek Cottage Cheese
Calories: 236

 DINNER
Ratatouille Cod
Calories: 411

TOTAL CALORIES: 1882

If you're a super health-conscious reader, remember that big, colourful salad bowls, fresh fruit smoothies, grains and fatty fish will all pack a SERIOUSLY nutritious punch!

In my experience, Japanese food will likely tick all of these boxes, so if you're looking for a healthy dinner date option, get down to your local sushi spot!

SHOPPING LIST ESSENTIALS

Protein

Eggs
———

0% Greek / plain
soy yoghurt (any)
———

Whey or vegan
protein powder
———

Chicken breasts
———

Salmon
(smoked and / or fillet)
———

Fillet steak
———

Prawns
———

Quorn (fillets or pieces)
———

Tofu pieces
———

Lunchmeat (lean ham /
wafer thin chicken /
turkey slices)
———

Carbohydrates

Oat sachets (any)
———

Plain cereal grains
(such as All Bran / Rice
Krispies / Puffed Oats)
———

Fruit (any)
———

Wholemeal bread (any)
———

Microwave rice (any)
———

Fresh pasta (any)
———

Starchy veg (such as
potatoes and parsnips)
———

Rice cakes (any)
———

Salad veg (such as
leafy greens, tomatoes,
cucumbers, peppers,
mushrooms and onions)
———

Legumes and pulses
———

Fats

Oil (any)
———

Eggs
———

Butter
———

Salmon
(smoked and / or fillet)
———

Avocado
———

Nuts (any)
———

Seeds (any)
———

Nut butter (any)
———

Nut milk (any)
———

Dark chocolate
(the darker the better!)
———

INDEX

A FINAL WORD

I hope this book has shown you that regardless of your goals you really can eat healthily and enjoy the odd 'treat'.

There really is no 'good' or 'bad' food...
There are simply higher calorie and lower calorie foods. More nutritious and less nutritious foods.

If you've spent all day eating low-calorie, leafy green salads, of course you can enjoy a cookie!

And that's what health is all about – finding a balance between what your body needs and what you enjoy.

You should never go too far one way or the other – it is just as unhealthy eating nothing but spinach as it is eating nothing but ice cream.

I urge you to understand your body and your brain, and to feed both what they need!

ACKNOWLEDGEMENTS

Thank you to my husband, James, for forcing me to meet with your literary agent when I had all but given up hope on a book deal... here we are at number FOUR! Thank you for pushing me to work harder and be better every single day. If I can inspire even 1% of the amount of people you have, I will die a VERY happy girl.

That leads me nicely on to thanking my incredible literary agent, Clare Hulton. It feels a bit odd calling an agent 'talented', but that's how I often find myself describing you to people. Talented, warm, funny and works her socks off for her authors. I am so happy to have you on side!

Thank you to Transworld for letting me write a fourth book! We have been through A LOT together now guys! Michelle Signore, Emma Burton and Becky Short – it is SUCH a joy to work with such clever, funny, hard-working women. I love all three of you to bits.

Thank you to Jo Roberts-Miller for doing all the nitty gritty dirty work that makes this book SO MUCH BETTER! You add so much value to the content of my books, which my readers then give me all the credit for. I salute you, Jo!

Thank you Emma and Alex Smith for making all my books look utterly FANTASTIC and keeping them as easy to read, understand and digest as humanly possible. You have a ridiculous amount of talent.

Thank you to Meera for being there for me on shoots through the good and the bad. You know more secrets than my friends and family, and I wouldn't have it any other way! You are such a tough cookie, I often find myself wondering 'What would Meera do?!' I love you girl.

Thank you Sam Riley for always making me laugh on shoot days and having a good old bitch with me about all the bad apples, ha!

Thank you to my family; my mum, dad, three brothers, three sisters-in-law, two nieces and one nephew. I live to make you all proud and I know I often fail at this when I've had some wine and get a bit gobby, but I look up to every single one of you so very much (yup, even the kids!).

Last but NEVER LEAST...

Thank you to my AMAZING audience who support me every single day without fail.

I hope there'll be a book five, but if there isn't, you know I'll keep ranting SOMEWHERE online, ha! Guys, you earned the BIGGEST thanks of them all.

THANK YOU SO MUCH.